Mediterranean Diet for Beginners

The Complete Guide - Healthy and Easy Mediterranean Diet Recipes for Weight Loss - Prevention of Cardiovascular Diseases - Everything You Need to Get Started – 7 Day Diet Meal Plan

Tina Cooper

ISBN: 9781096964131

Table of Content

Introduction 8

Chapter 1: Understanding the Mediterranean Diet 10

What is the Mediterranean Diet? 10

Understanding the Mediterranean Cuisine by the region 10

The Science Behind the Mediterranean Diet 14

Chapter 2: Living Healthier and Longer on the Mediterranean Diet 17

The Incredible Health Benefits of Following the Mediterranean Diet 17

A Delicious Path to Weight Loss 18

Chapter 3: Starting the Mediterranean Diet 21

Planning Your Mediterranean Diet 21

Simple Tips to Follow 22

Chapter 4: Eating on the Mediterranean Diet 23

What Should you Have on Your Plate? 23

Your Shopping Guide 23

Eating Out on the Mediterranean Diet 27

A Sample Seven Day Meal Plan 28

Chapter 5: Breakfast 29

Hearty Pear and Mango Smoothie 29

Lovely Eggplant Salad 31

Lovely Artichoke Frittata 33

Full Eggs in a Squash 35

The Great Barley Porridge 37

Cool Tomato and Dill Frittata 39

Hearty Strawberry and Rhubarb Smoothie 41
Colorful Bacon and Brie Omelette Wedges................... 43
Pearl Couscous Salad 45
Simple Coconut Porridge 48
Crumbled Feta and Scallions 50
Early Morning Quinoa Chicken Salad........................... 52
Gnocchi Ham Olives.. 54
Spicy Early Morning Seafood Risotto 56
Rocket Tomatoes and Mushroom Frittata.................... 58

Chapter 6: Lunch 60
Favorite Pepper Soup.. 60
The Mediterranean Tomato Soup 62
Authentic Yogurt and Cucumber Salad......................... 64
Delightful Pesto Pizza... 66
Linguine Dredged in Tomato Clam Sauce 68
Wild Mushrooms and Pork Chops 70
Mediterranean Lamb Chops 72
Mushroom and Beef Risotto 74
Broiled Mushrooms Burgers and Goat Cheese 76
Tuna and Potato Salad 78
Parmesan and Chicken Veggie 80
Mushroom and Pork Chops 82
Oven Roasted Garlic Chicken Thigh 84
Trout with Wilted Greens... 86

Chapter 7: Dinner 88
Simple Dinnertime Radish and Beet Salad.................. 88
Chicken and Artichoke Salad 90
Kidney Beans and Cilantro Meal.................................... 92

Caramelized Onion and Fennel Pizza 94
Lovely Baked Chicken 96
Herbed and Lamb Cutlets 98
Sweet Potato Curry... 100
Herbed Pork Tenderloin 102
Green Bean Stew 104
Mediterranean Roast Chicken.................................... 106
Honey Chicken 108
Lovingly Broiled Calamari 110
Broccoli and Tilapia Meal 112
Authentic "Medi" Tilapia... 114
Premium and Healthy Chicken Cacciatore 116
Heavenly Poached Salmon... 118

Chapter 8: Side Dishes 120
Summertime Vegetable Chicken Wraps 120
Premium Roasted Baby Potatoes...............................122
Tomato and Cherry Linguine 124
Mediterranean Zucchini Mushroom Pasta 126
Lemon and Garlic Fettucine.......................................128
Roasted Broccoli with Parmesan 130
Spinach and Feta Bread 132
Quick Zucchini Bowl 134
Healthy Basil Platter 136
Herbed Up Bruschetta 138
Homemade Almond Biscotti...................................... 140

Chapter 9: Dessert 142
Almond and Chocolate Butter Dip..............................142
Strawberry and Feta Delight......................................144

Simple Strawberry Yogurt Ice Cream 146

Pear with Honey Drizzles 148

Cherry and Olive Bites 150

Fluffed Up Chocolate Mousse 152

Chocolate Butter Dip 154

Mouthwatering Panna Cotta with Mixed Berry Compote 156

Grilled Peaches and Egyptian Dukkah with Blueberries 158

Lemon Mousse 160

Avocado Cool Dish 162

Icy Berry Popsicles 164

Spiced Up Mug Cake 166

Hearty Cashew and Almond Butter 168

Chapter 10: Snacks 170

Brussels Sprouts and Pistachios 170

Hearty Cucumber Soup 172

Spiced Up Kale Chips 174

Fresh Veggies with Hummus 176

Crazy Almond Crackers 178

Superb Stuffed Mushrooms 180

Flax and Almond Crunchies 182

Mashed Up Celeriac 184

Baked Feta and Spinach Meal 186

Easy Medi Kale 188

Black Bean Hummus 190

Strawberry and Feta Salad 192

Baked Falafel Dish 194

Conclusion **196**
© Copyright 2019 – Tina Cooper- All rights reserved. 197

Introduction

Recent studies indicate that in the United States and the Western Civilization in general, the primary cause of mortality is various forms of cardiac diseases, atherosclerosis and artery blockages.

While there are many synthetic and medicinal ways a person can help to cure themselves, prevention is always better than cure, right?

And that is exactly where the Mediterranean Diet comes in!

To keep things short and simple, the Mediterranean Diet is possibly one of the most unique diet programs available right now that focuses on keeping your heart healthy as opposed to trimming down your weight. Keep in mind though, that even if your target is to lose weight, the Mediterranean Diet will still help you to do that!

For those of you who are completely unfamiliar, the Mediterranean Diet basically follows the foods and lifestyle of people who live alongside the borders of the Mediterranean Sea, which includes France, Spain, Greece, and Italy.

The Mediterranean Diet focuses on consuming seafood, fish, vegetables and a good amount of olive oil while eliminating any processed food and even sugar that would cause harm to the health of your heart.

The Mediterranean Diet is possibly one of those rare food programs that asks you to not only rely on a diet but also incorporate a healthy lifestyle and well-rounded social activities to ultimately ensure that that you lead a prolonged and healthy life.

All of these small factors work together to make the Mediterranean Diet the number one choice for dieticians and nutritionists all around the world when it comes to improving your heart health!

And these are not just words. The American Heart Association has even boasted the Mediterranean Diet as being one of the best diets to help you improve your cardiac health.

That being said, the first few chapters of the book will help you to understand the basics of the Mediterranean Diet while the remaining chapters will walk you through some amazing recipes to inspire you for the future.

Chapter 1: Understanding the Mediterranean Diet

What is the Mediterranean Diet?

The Mediterranean Diet is possibly one of the most unique and "Off-Beat" diets out there in the market. While most diets tend to focus on trimming down your excess body weight, losing, the Mediterranean Diet takes things further and shifts its focus on trying to make you healthier. In particular, make your "Heart" healthier.

The core basics of the Mediterranean Diet are prepared and designed to include all of the basics of healthy eating and indirectly encourages an individual to further encourage a healthy lifestyle by choosing healthy ingredients and preparing heart-friendly meals.

To put it simply, the Mediterranean Diet puts a lot of emphasis on going after more and more green colored foods. On the other hand, you will be recommended to replace dairy products such as butter with other healthy oils such as olive oil and canola oil.

If things seem a little bit confusing right now, don't worry! We will be diving a little bit deeper into the core concepts of the Mediterranean Diet to help you understand the basics.

For now, let's first have a look at the origin of the Mediterranean Diet.

Understanding the Mediterranean Cuisine by the region

The Mediterranean Cuisine is a fascinating one as it incorporates all the traditional healthy foods and eating habits of people living in the countries that border the Mediterranean Sea.

This means you are looking at Greece, Spain, Italy and France.

The Mediterranean Diet actually has a really good amount of variation depending on the "region" you are looking at, which also alters the core definition to some extent.

However, the core of the diet always remains the same, and you will be asked to consume meals that are high in vegetables, legumes, fruit, beans, grains, olive oil, unsaturated and unsaturated fats.

The levels of meat and dairy products should be kept at low levels! That being said, below is a brief look into the various regions and the ingredients that they incorporate:

Morocco: Moroccan cooking uses an exotic mixture of flavors that focus on both sweet and savory accents. Moroccan foods have a strong flavor but are generally less spicy.

Common ingredients include:

- Cinnamon
- Cumin
- Dried Fruits
- Ginger
- Lemon
- Mint
- Paprika
- Parsley
- Saffron
- Turmeric
- Pepper

Spain: Regardless of what part of Spain you decide to consider, you can always count on a good dose of garlic and olive oil in the dishes. Spanish meals are often inspired by Arabic and Roman cuisine and emphasise fresh seafood.

Common ingredients include:

- Almonds
- Anchovies
- Cheese (Goat, Sheep, and Cow)
- Garlic
- Ham
- Honey
- Onions
- Olive Oil
- Oregano
- Rosemary
- Nuts
- Paprika
- Thyme

Southern Italy: Italian food is generally very rich and savory and has very strong flavored ingredients. Usually, tomato-based sauces and various types of spices are used as well.

Commonly used ingredients include:

- Anchovies
- Balsamic vinegar
- Basil
- Bay Leaf
- Parsley
- Mozzarella cheese
- Olive Oil
- Oregano
- Mushrooms
- Rosemary
- Sage
- Thyme

- Tomatoes

Greece: When it comes to Greek cooking, they try to focus on tangy and citrus flavors.

Common ingredients include:

- Basil
- Cucumbers
- Dill
- Feta cheese
- Fennel
- Honey
- Garlic
- Lemon
- Pepper
- Saffron
- Turmeric

The Science Behind the Mediterranean Diet

To understand the concept behind the Mediterranean Diet, you must learn to appreciate what is called a "Mediterranean Food Pyramid."

The Mediterranean Diet actually includes a very special balance of foods that exposes the body to a good amount of vitamins, minerals and anti-oxidants and a perfect balance of fatty acids.

However, as the pyramid dictates, the Mediterranean Diet doesn't really focus only on the food part.

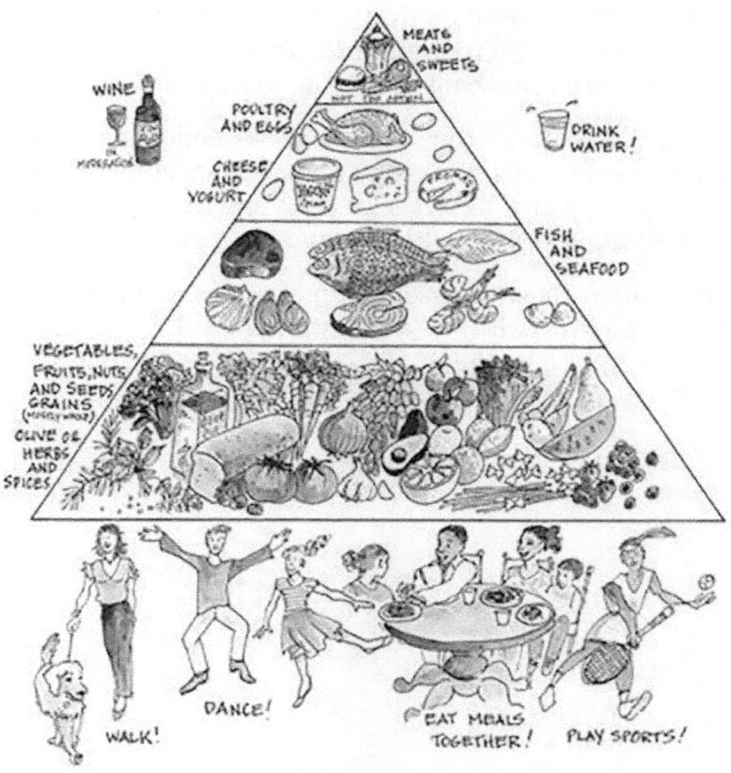

Rather, it also focuses on encouraging a healthy and joyful lifestyle to accompany the healthy food.

Following the Mediterranean diet and a healthy lifestyle would require you to have considered both your dietary and social aspects of life.

This means you should have time for rest, fun and socializing with folks that are close to you and keep some time aside for daily physical activities.

To tie everything up together, the Oldways Preservation and Exchange Trust came up with a simple and easy to follow chart known as the Mediterranean Food Guide Pyramid that is based on the dietary traditions of Greece and Southern Italy (1960s), which was a time when the rate of heart disease and cancer were at an all-time low.

As you can see from the diagram above, following a proper Mediterranean Diet will require you to focus on vegetables, whole grain, fruits, legumes, seafood and a little bit of meat, while eliminating unhealthy fat and processed food.

And perhaps most importantly, make sure to make enough time to have fun with your family and friends!

Chapter 2: Living Healthier and Longer on the Mediterranean Diet

As you can already tell, the Mediterranean Diet will take you on a path of becoming your healthier self!

The Incredible Health Benefits of Following the Mediterranean Diet

Just some of the awesome benefits that you will enjoy include:

- This particular diet will help you to lower chronic stress and help you relax.

- Since the Mediterranean Diet is centered around the consumption of fresh and healthy plants and healthy fats, it will help to improve longevity and make life longer. The core fat used in the Mediterranean Diet (The main source of fat in the Mediterranean Diet), is proven to lower levels of heart disease, cancer, Alzheimer's and so on.

- There is much evidence that shows how the Mediterranean Diet helps to prevent Parkinson's disease and improve your memory, which, in turn, helps to cure Alzheimer's and dementia as well. Healthy Fats coming from olive oil, nuts, and anti-inflammatory vegetables are well-known to improve your overall mental health

- Since you will be going on a low-sugar diet, it will help you stay safe from diabetes.

- According to the European Journal of Cancer Prevention, the biological mechanism that is associated with cancer prevention, have seen significant improvements in individuals who tend to follow a Mediterranean Diet, thanks to the balanced ratio of omega 6, omega 3 fatty acids and a good amount of fiber, polyphenols, antioxidants that come from olive oil, vegetables, fruit and wine. Due to this, the Mediterranean diet is also considered to be a natural cure for cancer by many.

- Since you will mostly be focusing on low-processed meals, the Mediterranean Diet will significantly help to cut down the consumption of artificial ingredients or ingredients that are packed with GMOs; it will ultimately help to improve the health of your heart and maintain good cholesterol.

- Various research has shown that the monosaturated fats and omega-3 rich foods that make up a large part of the Mediterranean Diet greatly reduce the possibility of heart diseases and improves your overall cardiovascular health. Olive oil also helps to control hypertension and reduces blood pressure.

A Delicious Path to Weight Loss

Despite the Mediterranean Diet primarily focusing on just keeping you healthy, the Mediterranean Diet can actually be used to lose a good amount of weight while not letting go of all the delicious meals that you so dearly love!

According to a recent study known as "PREDIMED," it has been shown that individuals who follow a Mediterranean Diet have put on the least amount of weight and have even lost weight in the long run.

A similar report was published in the NEW ENGLAND JOURNAL of MEDICINE that further solidified the concept that it is indeed possible to lose weight by following the Mediterranean Diet.

While following the diet will naturally help you lose weight, the following tips should further help to trim down your weight:

- Always try to eat your main meal as early as possible. It will prevent you from overeating later in the day.

- When considering your main course, try to keep it as veggie packed as possible and use olive oil for cooking. Veggie dishes are usually low in carbohydrates and will help you with your weight loss.

- Try to consume as much water as you possibly can and opt for tea, coffee, and wine in small amounts.

- Try not to overshoot the amount of olive oil that you consume. Even though it is healthy, it is still recommended that you maintain a good balance. Good advice is to keep your olive oil intake to about 3 tablespoons per day.

- As you can already tell, the Mediterranean Diet is not only comprised of cooking and eating, but it also encourages an individual to take some time off and exercise, walk or go out for a jogging session with your friends and family. This will greatly accelerate the rate at which you lose weight.

Chapter 3: Starting the Mediterranean Diet

It has been scientifically proven that the best and effective diets are mostly those that work with the body's natural process and internal environment to bring about the positive changes.

Planning Your Mediterranean Diet

Now that you know the basics of the Mediterranean Diet, you might be wondering how to start the diet, right?

Well, below is a very simple outline that you should follow to take the first steps in the Mediterranean Diet world. It will allow you to effortlessly dive into the world of the Mediterranean diet.

So,

- Always try to ensure that you have at least 5 portions of mixed vegetables and fruits every day.

- Always try to base your meals on starchy foods such as potatoes, rice, bread, and pasta, and when possible, opt for the whole grain versions.

- Eat beans, fish, eggs, pulses, meat and other types of protein but try to maintain a higher ratio of fish and seafood than regular meat.

- Always make sure that you go for healthy dairy alternatives such as low fat/low sugar versions .

- Make sure to drink about 6-8 glasses of water.

- If you have a meal that is high in salt, fat or sugar, make sure to have them in small amounts.

Simple Tips to Follow

When deciding to create your Smoothie, it is best if you can stick to the following ingredients as closely as possible for maximum benefits:

- Try to switch to a healthier oil as soon as possible.

- Make sure to go for more seafood and fish as opposed to red meat.

- Try to keep yourself well-fed with vegetables as much as you can.

- Try to keep your pantry packed with whole grain ingredients and consume them as much as possible.

- When you have the munchies for a snack, simply opt for nuts or regular fruits as opposed to other heavier ones.

- When you want to have something sweet, go for fruits and use them as desserts.

- Make sure to exercise as much as possible.

Chapter 4: Eating on the Mediterranean Diet

It has been scientifically proven that the best and effective diets are mostly the ones that work with the body's natural process and internal environment to bring about the positive changes.

What Should you Have on Your Plate?

By now, you should already have a good idea of what to eat on the Mediterranean diet, but just to summarize:

- You should try to include fruits, seeds, nuts, vegetables, potatoes, bread, whole grain, herbs, fish, spices, seafood liberally and keep them in your platter.

- Eggs, yogurt, cheese, and poultry should be eaten in moderation.

- Beef, pork and other red meats should be eaten rarely or as minimally as possible.

- Completely avoid processed meat, sugar, sweetened beverages and refined grains from reaching your plate.

But that's just a general idea, the next section elaborates the concept further.

Your Shopping Guide

Aside from knowing how to start your diet, you should also know a little bit about how to set-up your pantry.

What to go for

- All kinds of vegetables including tomatoes, kale, broccoli, spinach, cauliflower, Brussels sprouts, carrots, cucumbers, etc.
- All types of fruits such as orange, apple, banana, pears, grapes, dates, strawberries, figs, melons, peaches, etc.
- Nuts and seeds such as almonds, Macadamia, walnuts, cashews, sunflower seeds, pumpkin seeds, etc.
- Legumes such as beans, lentils, peas, pulses, chickpeas etc.
- Tubers such as yams, turnips, potatoes, sweet potatoes and so on
- Whole grains such as whole oats, rye, brown rice, corn, barley, buckwheat, whole wheat, whole grain pasta, and bread
- Fish and seafood such as sardines, salmon, tuna, shrimp, mackerel, oyster, crab, clams, mussels, etc.
- Poultry such as turkey, chicken, duck and more
- Eggs including duck, quail and chicken eggs
- Dairy such as cheese, Greek yogurt, etc.
- Herbs and spices such as mint, basil, garlic, rosemary, cinnamon, sage, pepper, etc.
- Healthy fats and oil such as extra virgin olive oil, avocado oil, olives, etc.

What to avoid

- Foods with added sugar such as soda, ice cream, candies, table sugar, etc.

- Refined grains such as white bread or pasta made with refined wheat
- Margarine and similar processed foods that contain Trans Fats
- Refined oil such as cottonseed oil, soybean oil, etc.
- Processed meat such as hot dogs, processed sausages and so on
- Highly processed food with labels such as "Low-Fat" or "Diet" or anything that is not natural

Oils to know about

The Mediterranean Diet emphasizes healthy oils. The following are some of the oils that you might want to consider.

Coconut Oil: When it comes to high heat cooking, coconut oil is the best with over 90 of the fatty acids being saturated, which makes it very resistant to heat. This particular oil is semi-solid at room temperature and can be used for months without it turning rancid.

This particular oil also has a lot of health benefits! Since this oil is rich in a fatty acid known as Lauric Acid, it can help to improve cholesterol levels and kill various pathogens.

Extra-Virgin Olive Oil: Olive Oils are renowned worldwide for being one of the healthiest oils, and this is exactly why the Mediterranean Diet uses this oil as its key ingredient.

Some recent studies have shown that olive oil can even help to improve health biomarkers such as increasing the HDL cholesterol and lowering the amount of bad LDL cholesterol.

Avocado Oil: The composition of Avocado oil is very similar to olive oil and as such, it holds similar health benefits. It can be used for many purposes as an alternative for olive oil (Such as cooking).

Healthy salt alternatives

Asides from replacing healthy oils, the Mediterranean Diet will also ask you to opt for healthy salt alternatives as well. Below are some that you might want to consider.

Sunflower Seeds

Sunflower seeds are excellent and give a nutty and sweet flavor.

Fresh Squeezed Lemon

Lemon is believed to a be a nice hybrid between citron and bitter orange. These are packed with Vitamin C, which helps to neutralize damaging free radicals from the system.

Onion Powder

Onion powder is a dehydrated ground spice made from onion bulb, which is mostly used as a seasoning and is a fine salt alternative.

Black Pepper Powder

The black pepper powder is also a salt alternative that is native to India. Use it by grinding whole peppercorns!

Cinnamon

Cinnamon is very well-known as a savory spice, and two varieties are available: Ceylon and Chinese. Both of them sport a kind of sharp, warm and sweet flavor.

Flavored Vinegar

Fruit infused vinegar or flavored vinegar as we call it in our book are mixtures of vinegar that are combined with fruits in order to give a nice flavor. These are excellent ingredients to add a bit of flavor to meals without salt. Experimentation might be required to find the perfect fruit blend for you.

As for the process of making the vinegar:

- Wash your fruits and slice them well
- Place ½ a cup of your fruit in a mason jar
- Top them up with white wine vinegar (or balsamic vinegar)
- Allow them to sit for 2 weeks or so
- Strain and use as needed

Eating Out on the Mediterranean Diet

Initially, it might seem a little bit confusing, but eating out at a restaurant while on a Mediterranean Diet is actually pretty easy. Just follow the steps below:

- Try to ensure that you choose seafood or fish as the main dish of your meal
- When ordering, try to make a special request and ask the restaurant to fry their food using extra virgin olive oil
- Ask for only whole-grain based ingredients if possible
- If possible, try to read the menu of the restaurant before going there
- Try to have a simple snack before you go to the restaurant; this will help prevent you from overeating

A Sample Seven Day Meal Plan

Week 1	Sunday	Monday	Tuesday	Wednesday	Thursday	Friday	Saturday
Breakfast	Early Morning Quinoa Chicken Salad	Colorful Bacon and Brie Omelet Wedges	Cool Tomato and Dill Frittata	Early Morning Quinoa Chicken Salad	Colorful Bacon and Brie Omelet Wedges	Cool Tomato and Dill Frittata	Lovely Eggplant Salad
Lunch	Lovely Artichoke Frittata	Full Eggs in Corn	Hearty Cucumber Soup	Lovely Artichoke Frittata	Full Eggs in Corn	Hearty Cucumber Soup	Crumbled Feta and Scallions
Dinner	Lovely Baked Chicken	Broccoli Tilapia	Heavenly Poached Salmon	Lovely Baked Chicken	Broccoli Tilapia	Heavenly Poached Salmon	Lovely Baked Chicken

Chapter 5: Breakfast
Hearty Pear and Mango Smoothie

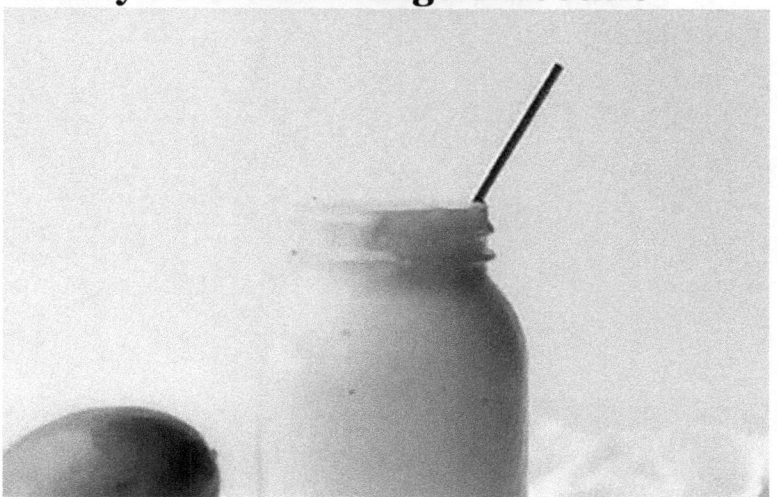

Serving: 1

Prep Time: 10 minutes

Cook Time: nil

Ingredients

- 1 ripe mango, cored and chopped
- ½ mango, peeled, pitted and chopped
- 1 cup kale, chopped
- ½ cup plain Greek yogurt
- 2 ice cubes

How To

1. Add pear, mango, yogurt, kale, and mango to a blender and puree.
2. Add ice and blend until you have a smooth texture.
3. Serve and enjoy!

Nutrition (Per Serving)

- Calories: 293
- Fat: 8g
- Carbohydrates: 53g
- Protein: 8g

Lovely Eggplant Salad

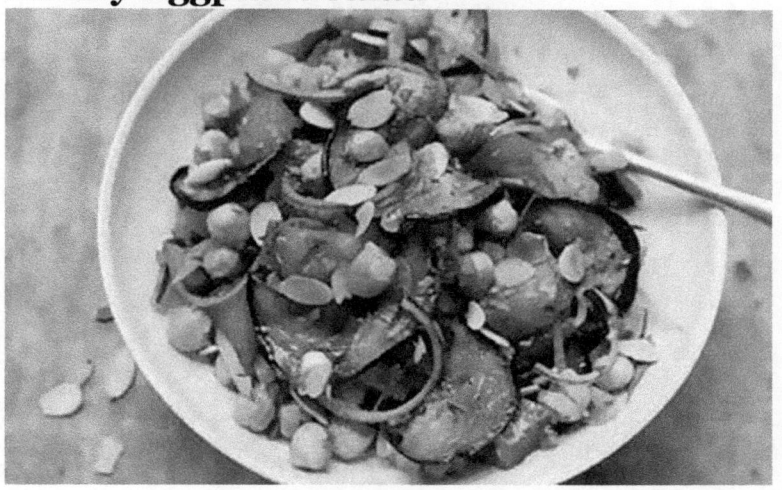

Serving: 8

Prep Time: 20 minutes

Cook Time: 15 minutes

Ingredients

- 1 large eggplant, washed and cubed
- 1 tomato, seeded and chopped
- 1 small onion, diced
- 2 tablespoons parsley, chopped
- 2 tablespoons extra virgin olive oil
- 2 tablespoons distilled white vinegar
- ½ cup feta cheese, crumbled
- Salt as needed

How To

1. Pre-heat your outdoor grill to medium-high.
2. Pierce the eggplant a few times using a knife/fork.
3. Cook the eggplants on your grill for about 15 minutes until they are charred.

4. Keep it on the side and allow them to cool.
5. Remove the skin from the eggplant and dice the pulp.
6. Transfer the pulp to a mixing bowl and add parsley, onion, tomato, olive oil, feta cheese and vinegar.
7. Mix well and chill for 1 hour.
8. Season with salt and enjoy!

Nutrition (Per Serving)

- Calories: 99
- Fat: 7g
- Carbohydrates: 7g
- Protein: 3.4g

Lovely Artichoke Frittata

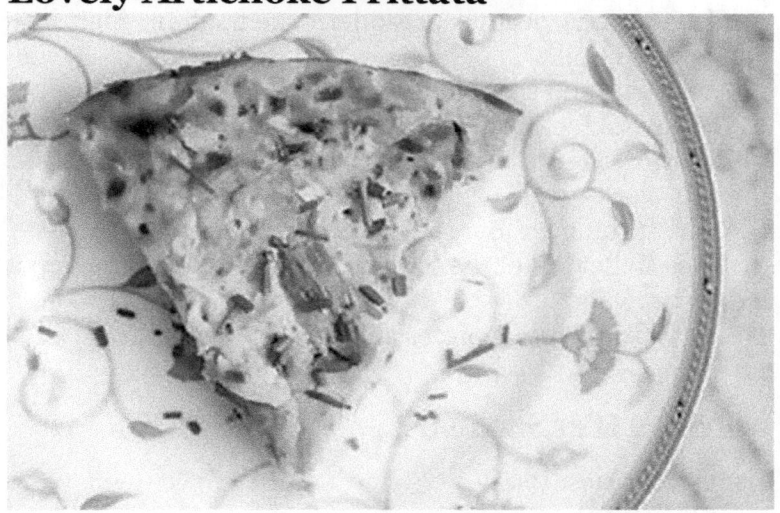

Serving: 4

Prep Time: 5 minutes

Cook Time: 10 minutes

Ingredients

- 8 large eggs
- ¼ cup Asiago cheese, grated
- 1 tablespoon fresh basil, chopped
- 1 teaspoon fresh oregano, chopped
- Pinch of salt
- 1 teaspoon extra virgin olive oil
- 1 teaspoon garlic, minced
- 1 cup canned artichokes, drained
- 1 tomato, chopped

How To

1. Pre-heat your oven to broil.
2. Take a medium bowl and whisk in eggs, Asiago cheese, oregano, basil, sea salt and pepper.

3. Blend in a bowl.
4. Place a large ovenproof skillet over medium-high heat and add olive oil.
5. Add garlic and sauté for 1 minute.
6. Remove skillet from heat and pour in egg mix.
7. Return skillet to heat and sprinkle artichoke hearts and tomato over eggs.
8. Cook frittata without stirring for 8 minutes.
9. Place skillet under the broiler for 1 minute until the top is lightly browned.
10. Cut frittata into 4 pieces and serve.
11. Enjoy!

Nutrition (Per Serving)

- Calories: 199
- Fat: 13g
- Carbohydrates: 5g
- Protein: 16g

Full Eggs in a Squash

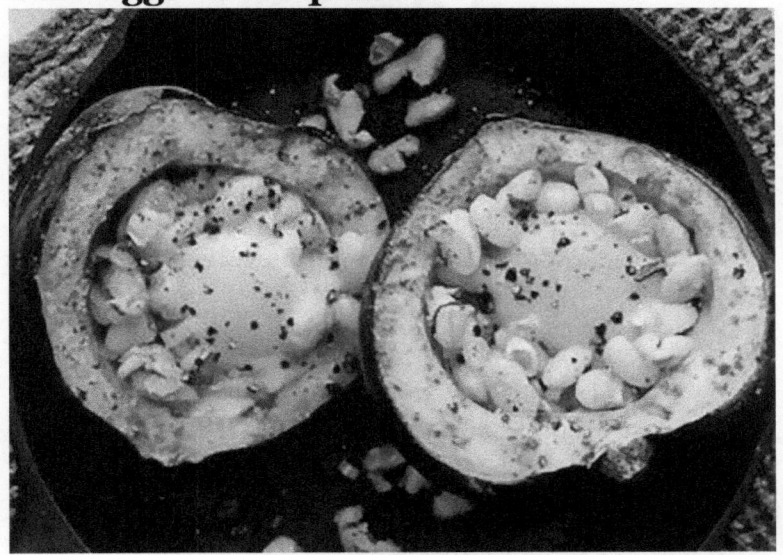

Serving: 5

Prep Time: 10 minutes

Cook Time: 20 minutes

Ingredients

- 2 acorn squash
- 6 whole eggs
- 2 tablespoons extra virgin olive oil
- Salt and pepper as needed
- 5-6 pitted dates
- 8 walnut halves
- A fresh bunch of parsley

How To

1. Pre-heat your oven to 375 degrees Fahrenheit.
2. Slice squash crosswise and prepare 3 slices with holes.

3. While slicing the squash, make sure that each slice has a measurement of ¾ inch thickness.
4. Remove the seeds from the slices.
5. Take a baking sheet and line it with parchment paper.
6. Transfer the slices to your baking sheet and season them with salt and pepper.
7. Bake in your oven for 20 minutes.
8. Chop the walnuts and dates on your cutting board .
9. Take the baking dish out of the oven and drizzle slices with olive oil.
10. Crack an egg into each of the holes in the slices and season with pepper and salt.
11. Sprinkle the chopped walnuts on top.
12. Bake for 10 minutes more.
13. Garnish with parsley and add maple syrup.
14. Enjoy!

Nutrition (Per Serving)

- Calories: 198
- Fat: 12g
- Carbohydrates: 17g
- Protein: 8g

The Great Barley Porridge

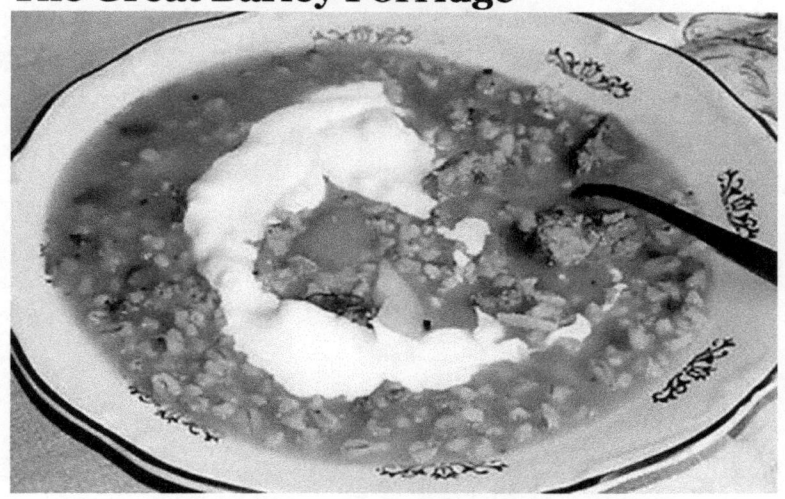

Serving: 4

Prep Time: 5 minutes

Cook Time: 25 minutes

Ingredients

- 1 cup barley
- 1 cup wheat berries
- 2 cups unsweetened almond milk
- 2 cups water
- ½ cup blueberries
- ½ cup pomegranate seeds
- ½ cup hazelnuts, toasted and chopped
- ¼ cup honey

How To

1. Take a medium saucepan and place it over medium-high heat.
2. Place barley, almond milk, wheat berries, water and bring to a boil.

3. Reduce the heat to low and simmer for 25 minutes.
4. Divide amongst serving bowls and top each serving with 2 tablespoons blueberries, 2 tablespoons pomegranate seeds, 2 tablespoons hazelnuts, 1 tablespoon honey.
5. Serve and enjoy!

Nutrition (Per Serving)

- Calories: 295
- Fat: 8g
- Carbohydrates: 56g
- Protein: 6g

Cool Tomato and Dill Frittata

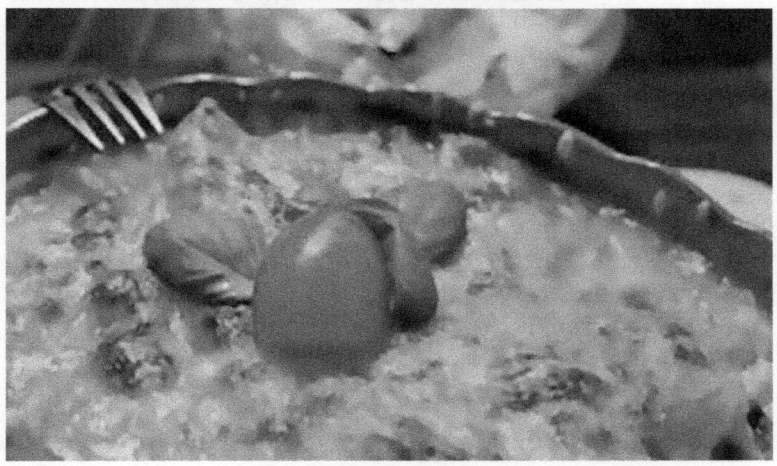

Serving: 4

Prep Time: 5 minutes

Cook Time: 10 minutes

Ingredients

- 2 tablespoons olive oil
- 1 medium onion, chopped
- 1 teaspoon garlic, minced
- 2 medium tomatoes, chopped
- 6 large eggs
- ½ cup half and half
- ½ cup feta cheese, crumbled
- ¼ cup dill weed
- Salt as needed
- Ground black pepper as needed

How To

1. Pre-heat your oven to a temperature of 400 degrees Fahrenheit.

2. Take a large sized ovenproof pan and heat up your olive oil over medium-high heat.
3. Toss in the onion, garlic, tomatoes and stir fry them for 4 minutes.
4. While they are being cooked, take a bowl and beat together your eggs, half and half cream and season the mix with some pepper and salt.
5. Pour the mixture into the pan with your vegetables and top it with crumbled feta cheese and dill weed.
6. Cover it with the lid and let it cook for 3 minutes.
7. Place the pan inside your oven and let it bake for 10 minutes .
8. Serve hot.

Nutrition (Per Serving)

- Calories: 191
- Fat: 15g
- Carbohydrates: 6g
- Protein: 9g

Hearty Strawberry and Rhubarb Smoothie

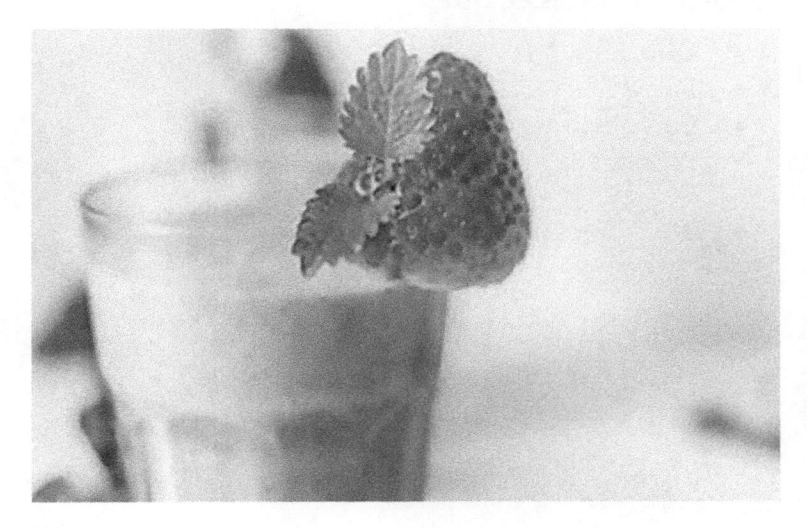

Serving: 1

Prep Time: 5 minutes

Cook Time: 3 minutes

Ingredients

- 1 rhubarb stalk, chopped
- 1 cup fresh strawberries, sliced
- ½ cup plain Greek strawberries
- Pinch of ground cinnamon
- 3 ice cubes

How To

1. Take a small saucepan and fill with water over high heat.
2. Bring to boil and add rhubarb, boil for 3 minutes.
3. Drain and transfer to blender.
4. Add strawberries, honey, yogurt, cinnamon and pulse mixture until smooth.

5. Add ice cubes and blend until thick with no lumps.
6. Pour into glass and enjoy chilled.

Nutrition (Per Serving)

- Calories: 295
- Fat: 8g
- Carbohydrates: 56g
- Protein: 6g

Colorful Bacon and Brie Omelette Wedges

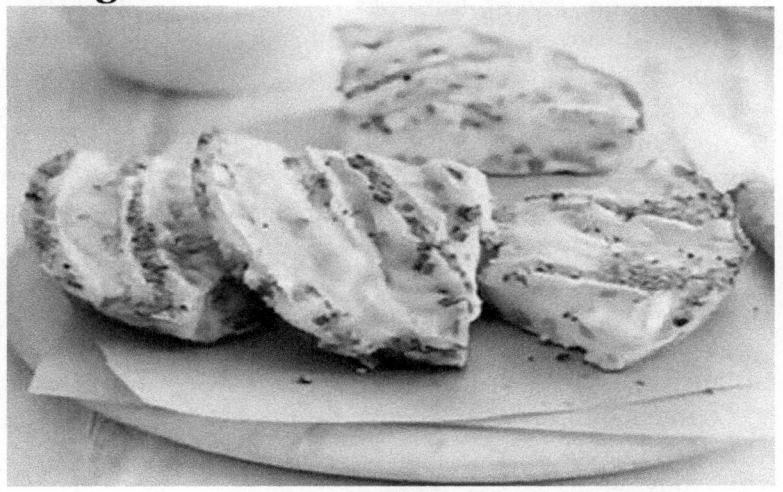

Serving: 6

Prep Time: 10 minutes

Cook Time: 10 minutes

Ingredients

- 2 tablespoons olive oil
- 7 ounces smoked bacon
- 6 beaten eggs
- Small bunch chives, snipped
- 3 ½ ounces brie, sliced
- 1 teaspoon red wine vinegar
- 1 teaspoon Dijon mustard
- 1 cucumber, halved, deseeded and sliced diagonally
- 7 ounces radish, quartered

How To

1. Turn your grill on and set it to high.

2. Take a small-sized pan and add 1 teaspoon of oil, allow the oil to heat up.
3. Add lardons and fry until crisp.
4. Drain the lardon on kitchen paper.
5. Take another non-sticky cast iron frying pan and place it over grill, heat 2 teaspoons of oil.
6. Add lardons, eggs, chives, ground pepper to the frying pan.
7. Cook on LOW until they are semi-set.
8. Carefully lay brie on top and grill until the Brie sets and is a golden texture .
9. Remove it from the pan and cut up into wedges.
10. Take a small bowl and create dressing by mixing olive oil, mustard, vinegar and seasoning.
11. Add cucumber to the bowl and mix, serve alongside the Omelette wedges.
12. Enjoy!

Nutrition (Per Serving)

- Calories: 35
- Fat: 31g
- Carbohydrates: 3g
- Protein: 25g

Pearl Couscous Salad

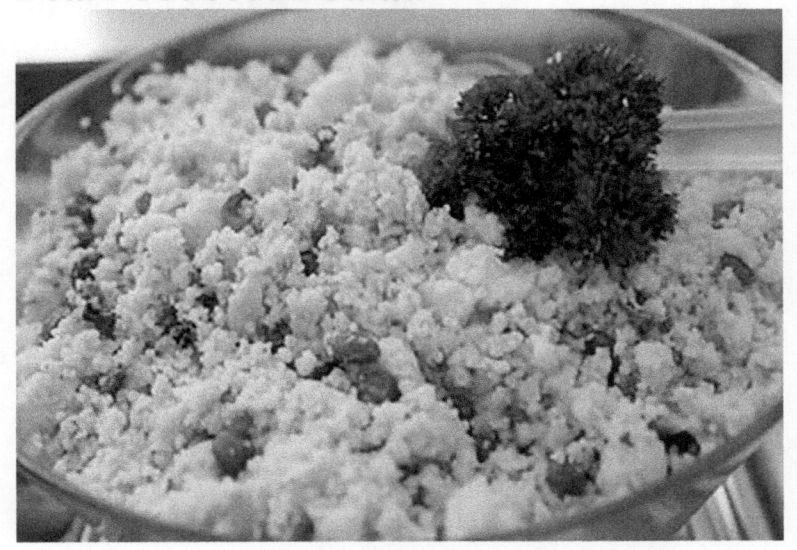

Serving: 6

Prep Time: 15 minutes

Cook Time: 0 minutes

Ingredients

For Lemon Dill Vinaigrette

- Juice of 1 large sized lemon
- 1/3 cup of extra virgin olive oil
- 1 teaspoon of dill weed
- 1 teaspoon of garlic powder
- Salt as needed
- Pepper

For Israeli Couscous

- 2 cups of Pearl Couscous
- Extra virgin olive oil
- 2 cups of halved grape tomatoes

- Water as needed
- 1/3 cup of finely chopped red onions
- ½ of a finely chopped English cucumber
- 15 ounces of chickpeas
- 14 ounce can of artichoke hearts (roughly chopped up)
- ½ cup of pitted Kalamata olives
- 15-20 pieces of fresh basil leaves, roughly torn and chopped up
- 3 ounces of fresh baby mozzarella

How To

1. Prepare the vinaigrette by taking a bowl and add the ingredients listed under vinaigrette.
2. Mix them well and keep aside.
3. Take a medium-sized heavy pot and place it over medium heat.
4. Add 2 tablespoons of olive oil and allow it to heat up.
5. Add couscous and keep cooking until golden brown.
6. Add 3 cups of boiling water and cook the couscous according to the package instructions.
7. Once done, drain in a colander and keep aside.
8. Take another large-sized mixing bowl and add the remaining ingredients except the cheese and basil.
9. Add the cooked couscous and basil to the mix and mix everything well.
10. Give the vinaigrette a nice stir and whisk it into the couscous salad.
11. Mix well.
12. Adjust the seasoning as required.
13. Add mozzarella cheese.
14. Garnish with some basil.
15. Enjoy!

Nutrition (Per Serving)

- Calories: 393

- Fat: 13g
- Carbohydrates: 57g
- Protein: 13g

Simple Coconut Porridge

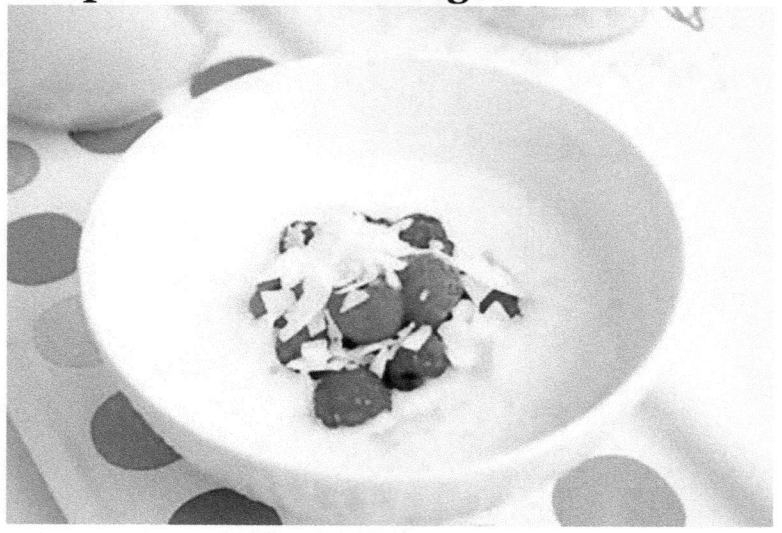

Serving: 6

Prep Time: 15 minutes

Cook Time: Nil

Ingredients

- Powdered erythritol as needed
- 1 ½ cups almond milk, unsweetened
- 2 tablespoons vanilla protein powder
- 3 tablespoons Golden Flaxseed meal
- 2 tablespoons coconut flour

How To

16. Take a bowl and mix in flaxseed meal, protein powder, coconut flour and mix well.
17. Add mix to saucepan (placed over medium heat).
18. Add almond milk and stir, let the mixture thicken.
19. Add your desired amount of sweetener and serve.
20. Enjoy!

Nutrition (Per Serving)

- Calories: 259
- Fat: 13g
- Carbohydrates: 5g
- Protein: 16g

Crumbled Feta and Scallions

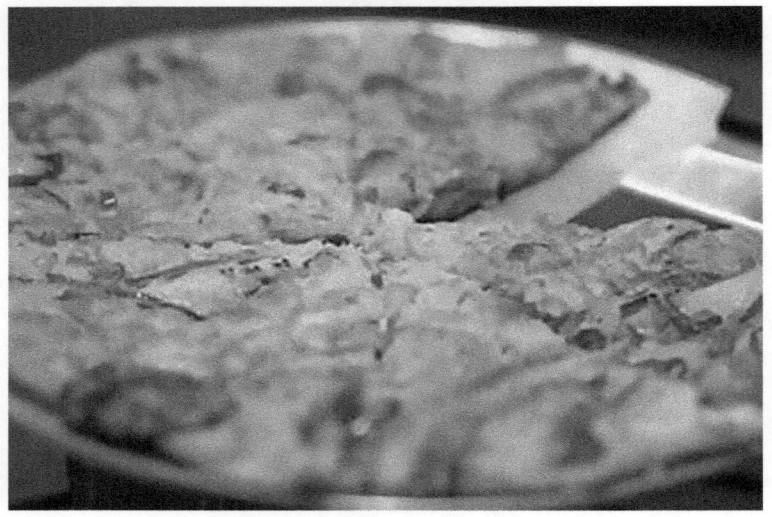

Serving: 12

Prep Time: 5 minutes

Cook Time: 15 minutes

Ingredients

- 2 tablespoon of unsalted butter (replace with canola oil for full effect)
- ½ cup of chopped up scallions
- 1 cup of crumbled feta cheese
- 8 large sized eggs
- 2/3 cup of milk
- ½ teaspoon of dried Italian seasoning
- Salt as needed
- Freshly ground black pepper as needed
- Cooking oil spray

How To

1. Pre-heat your oven to 400 degrees Fahrenheit.

2. Take a 3-4 ounce muffin pan and grease with cooking oil.
3. Take a non-stick pan and place it over medium heat.
4. Add butter and allow the butter to melt.
5. Add half of the scallions and stir fry.
6. Keep them to the side.
7. Take a medium-sized bowl and add eggs, Italian seasoning and milk and whisk well.
8. Add the stir fried scallions and feta cheese and mix.
9. Season with pepper and salt .
10. Pour the mix into the muffin tin.
11. Transfer the muffin tin to your oven and bake for 15 minutes.
12. Serve with a sprinkle of scallions.
13. Enjoy!

Nutrition(Per Serving)

- Calories: 106
- Fat: 8g
- Carbohydrates: 2g
- Protein: 7g

Early Morning Quinoa Chicken Salad

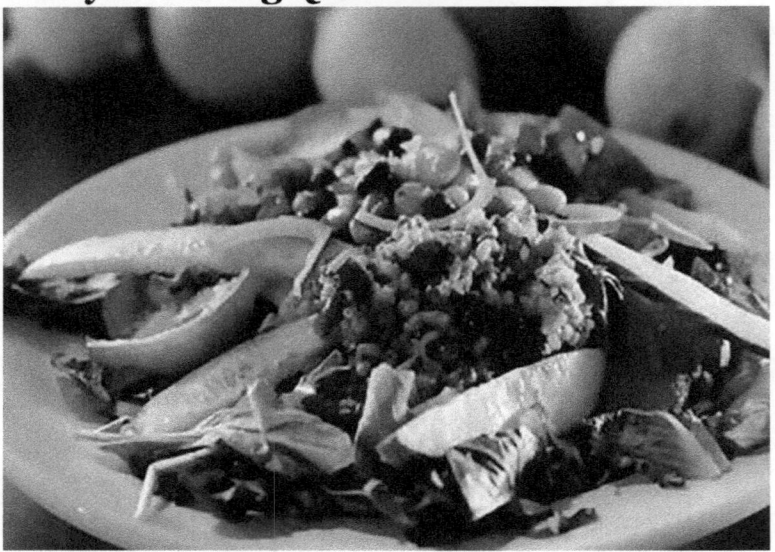

Serving: 8

Prep Time: 15 minutes

Cook Time: 20 minutes

Ingredients

- 2 cups of water
- 2 cubes of chicken bouillon
- 1 smashed garlic clove
- 1 cup of uncooked quinoa
- 2 large sized chicken breast cut up into bite-sized portions and cooked
- 1 large sized diced red onion
- 1 large sized green bell pepper
- ½ cup of Kalamata olives
- ½ cup of crumbled feta cheese
- ¼ cup of chopped up parsley
- ¼ cup of chopped up fresh chives

- ½ teaspoon of salt
- 1 tablespoon of balsamic vinegar
- ¼ cup of olive oil

How To

1. Take a saucepan and bring your water, garlic and bouillon cubes to a boil.
2. Stir in quinoa and reduce the heat to medium low.
3. Simmer for about 15-20 minutes until the quinoa has absorbed all the water and is tender.
4. Discard your garlic cloves and scrape the quinoa into a large sized bowl.
5. Gently stir in the cooked chicken breast, bell pepper, onion, feta cheese, chives, salt and parsley into your quinoa.
6. Drizzle some lemon juice, olive oil and balsamic vinegar.
7. Stir everything until mixed well.
8. Serve warm and enjoy!

Nutrition(Per Serving)

- Calories: 99
- Fat: 7g
- Carbohydrates: 7g
- Protein:3.4g

Gnocchi Ham Olives

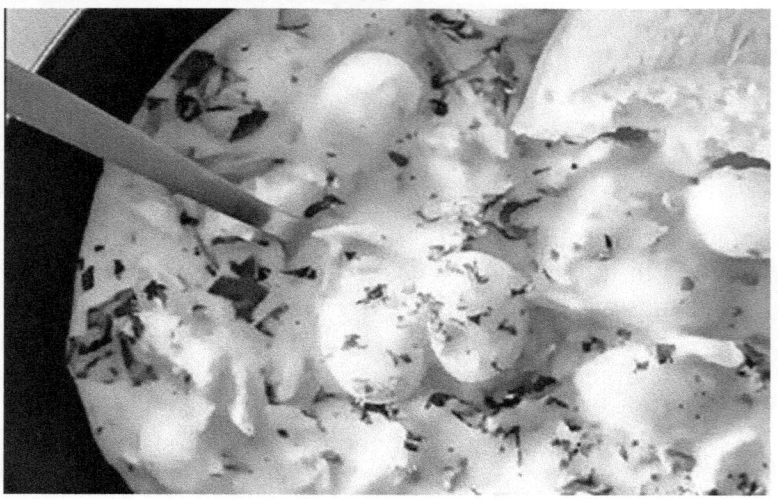

Prep Time: 5 minutes

Cooking Time: 15 minutes

Serving: 4

Ingredients

- 2 tablespoons of olive oil
- 1 medium-sized onion chopped up
- 3 minced cloves of garlic
- 1 medium-sized red pepper completely deseeded and finely chopped
- 1 cup of tomato puree
- 2 tablespoons of tomato paste
- 1 pound of gnocchi
- 1 cup of coarsely chopped turkey ham
- ½ cup of sliced pitted olives
- 1 teaspoon of Italian seasoning
- Salt as needed
- Freshly ground black pepper
- Bunch of fresh basil leaves

How To

1. Take a medium-sized sauce pan and place over medium-high heat.
2. Pour some olive oil and heat it up.
3. Toss in the bell pepper, onion and garlic and sauté for 2 minutes.
4. Pour in the tomato puree, gnocchi, tomato paste and add the turkey ham, Italian seasoning and olives.
5. Simmer the whole mix for 15 minutes, making sure to stir from time to time.
6. Season the mix with some pepper and salt.
7. Once done, transfer the mix to a dish and garnish with some basil leaves.
8. Serve hot and have fun.

Nutrition

- Calories: 335
- Fat: 12g
- Carbohydrates: 45g
- Protein: 15g

Spicy Early Morning Seafood Risotto

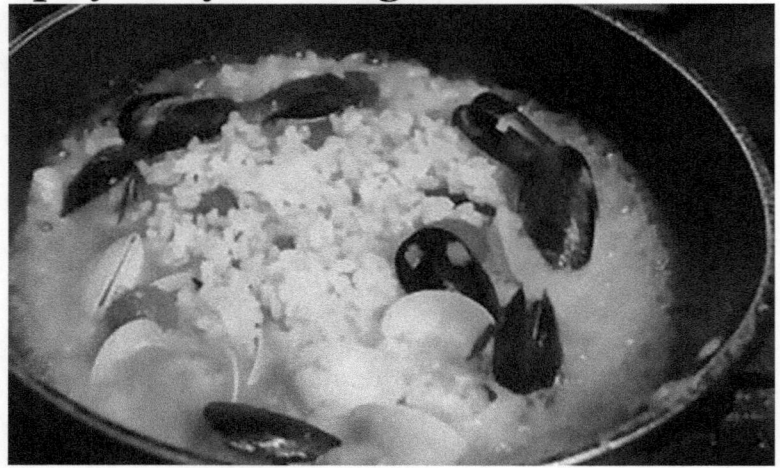

Prep Time: 5 minutes

Cooking Time: 15 minutes

Serving: 4

Ingredients

- 3 cups of clam juice
- 2 cups of water
- 2 tablespoons of olive oil
- 1 medium-sized chopped up onion
- 2 minced cloves of garlic
- 1 ½ cups of Arborio Rice
- ½ cup of dry white wine
- 1 teaspoon of Saffron
- ½ teaspoon of ground cumin
- ½ teaspoon of paprika
- 1 pound of marinara seafood mix
- Salt as needed
- Ground pepper as needed

How To

1. Place a saucepan over high heat and pour in your clam juice with water and bring the mixture to a boil.
2. Remove the heat.
3. Take a heavy bottomed saucepan and stir fry your garlic and onion in oil over medium heat until a nice fragrance comes off.
4. Add in the rice and keep stirring for 2-3 minutes until the rice has been fully covered with the oil.
5. Pour the wine and then add the saffron.
6. Keep stirring constantly until it is fully absorbed.
7. Add in the cumin, clam juice, paprika mixture 1 cup at a time, making sure to keep stirring it from time to time.
8. Cook the rice for 20 minutes until perfect.
9. Finally, add the seafood marinara mix and cook for another 5-7 minutes.
10. Season with some pepper and salt.
11. Transfer the meal to a serving dish.
12. Serve hot.

Nutrition

- Calories: 386
- Fat: 7g
- Carbohydrates: 55g
- Protein: 21g

Rocket Tomatoes and Mushroom Frittata

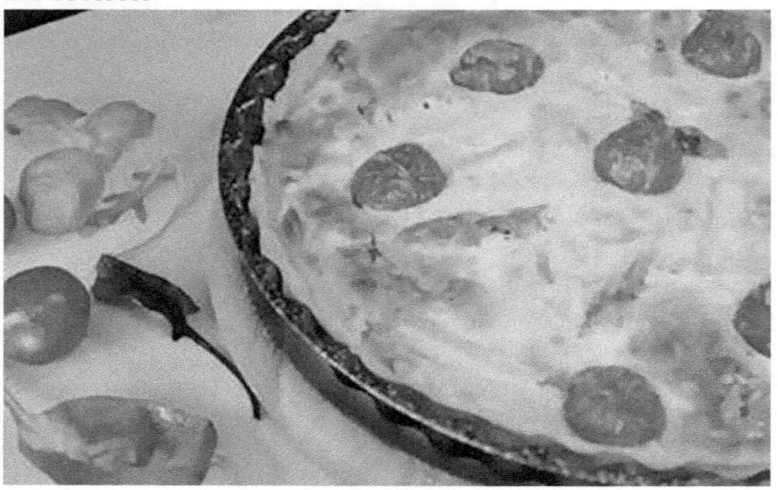

Serving: 4

Prep Time: 5 minutes

Cook Time: 15 minutes

Ingredients

- 2 tablespoons of butter (replace with canola oil for full effect)
- 1 chopped up medium-sized onion
- 2 minced cloves of garlic
- 1 cup of coarsely chopped baby rocket tomato
- 1 cup of sliced button mushrooms
- 6 large pieces of eggs
- ½ cup of skim milk
- 1 teaspoon of dried rosemary
- Salt as needed
- Ground black pepper as needed

How To

1. Pre-heat your oven to 400 degrees Fahrenheit.
2. Take a large oven-proof pan and place it over medium-heat.
3. Heat up some oil.
4. Stir fry your garlic, onion for about 2 minutes.
5. Add the mushroom, rosemary and rockets and cook for 3 minutes.
6. Take a medium-sized bowl and beat your eggs alongside the milk.
7. Season it with some salt and pepper.
8. Pour the egg mixture into your pan with the vegetables and sprinkle some Parmesan.
9. Reduce the heat to low and cover with the lid.
10. Let it cook for 3 minutes.
11. Transfer the pan into your oven and bake for 10 minutes until fully settled.
12. Reduce the heat to low and cover with your lid.
13. Let it cook for 3 minutes.
14. Transfer the pan into your oven and then bake for another 10 minutes.
15. Serve hot.

Nutrition(Per Serving)

- Calories: 189
- Fat: 13g
- Carbohydrates: 6g
- Protein: 12g

Chapter 6: Lunch
Favorite Pepper Soup

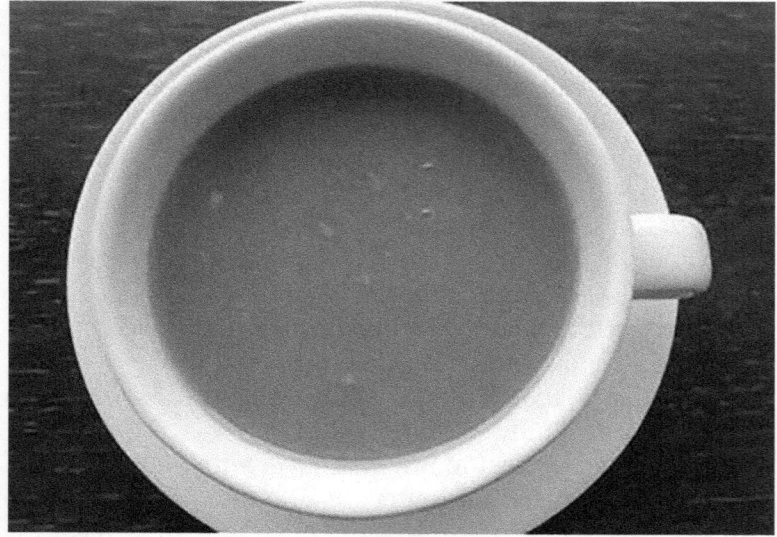

Serving: 6

Prep Time: 5 minutes

Cook Time: 30 minutes

Ingredients

- 1 pound lean ground beef
- 1 onion, chopped
- 1 large green pepper, chopped
- 2 garlic cloves, minced
- 1 large tomato, chopped
- 2 tablespoons tomato paste
- 2 tablespoons all-purpose flour
- ¼ cup uncooked rice
- 2 tablespoons fresh parsley, chopped
- 4 cups beef broth
- 2 tablespoons olive oil

- Salt and pepper as needed

How To

1. Take a large-sized pot and place it over medium heat.
2. Add oil and allow the oil to heat up.
3. Add flour and keep whisking until you have a thick paste.
4. Keep whisking for 3-4 minutes more while it bubbles and begins to thin.
5. Add chopped onion and sauté for 3-4 minutes.
6. Stir in tomato paste and beef.
7. Take a wooden spoon and stir to break the ground beef.
8. Cook for 5 minutes.
9. Add garlic, pepper and chopped tomatoes.
10. Mix well and combine.
11. Add broth and bring the mix to a light boil, reduce the heat to low and simmer for 30 minutes.
12. Add rice, parsley and cook for 15 minutes.
13. Once it has a nice soup-like consistency, serve with garnish of parsley.
14. Enjoy!

Nutrition (Per Serving)

- Calories: 162
- Fat: 3g
- Carbohydrates: 12g
- Protein: 21g

The Mediterranean Tomato Soup

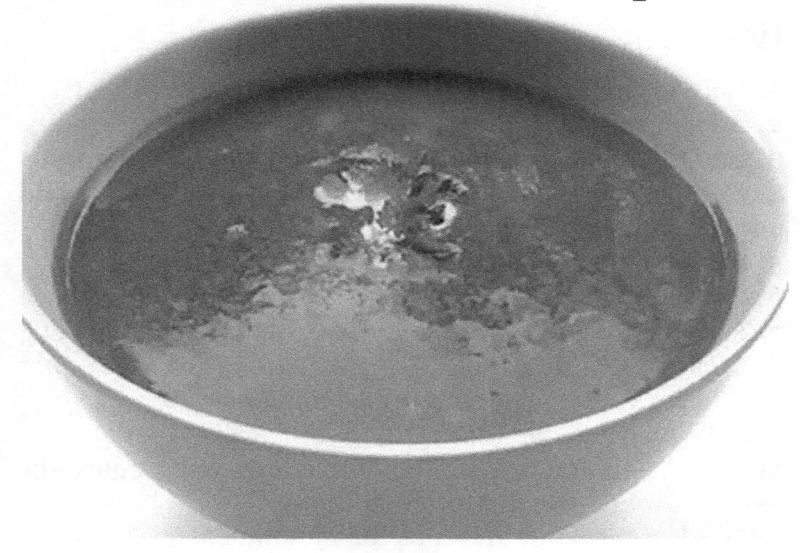

Serving: 6

Prep Time: 5 minutes

Cook Time: 25 minutes

Ingredients

- 4 tablespoons olive oil
- 2 medium yellow onion, thinly sliced
- 1 teaspoon salt
- 2 teaspoons curry powder
- 1 teaspoon red curry powder
- 1 teaspoon ground coriander
- 1 teaspoon ground cumin
- 1 can (15 ounces) Roma tomatoes, diced
- 1 can (28 ounce) plum tomatoes, diced
- 5 ½ cups water
- 1 can (14 ounces) coconut milk

- Coconut brown rice, lemon wedges, fresh thyme, etc. as extra mix-ins

How To

1. Take a medium-sized pan and add oil.
2. Place it over medium heat and allow it to heat up.
3. Add onions and salt and cook for about 10-12 minutes until browned .
4. Stir in curry powder, coriander, red pepper flakes, cumin and cook for 30 seconds.
5. Make sure to keep stirring it well.
6. Add tomatoes alongside the juice and 5 ½ cups of water (or broth if you prefer).
7. Simmer the mixture for 15 minutes .
8. Take an immersion blender and puree the mixture until a soupy consistency is achieved.
9. Enjoy as it is, or add some extra add-ins for a more flavorful experience.

Nutrition (Per Serving)

- Calories: 74
- Fat: 0.7g
- Carbohydrates: 16g
- Protein: 2g

Authentic Yogurt and Cucumber Salad

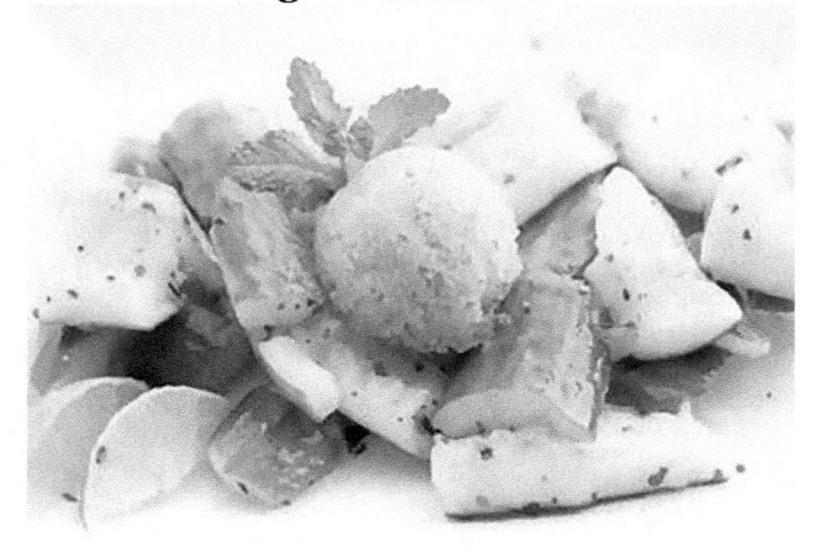

Serving: 4

Prep Time: 10 minutes

Cook Time: nil

Ingredients

- 5-6 small cucumbers, peeled and diced
- 1 (8 ounces) container plain Greek yogurt
- 2 garlic cloves, minced
- 1 tablespoon fresh mint, minced
- 1 teaspoon dried oregano
- Sea salt and fresh black pepper

How To

1. Take a large bowl and add cucumbers, garlic, yogurt, mint, and oregano.
2. Season with salt and pepper.
3. Refrigerate the salad for 1 hour and serve.

4. Enjoy!

<u>Nutrition (Per Serving)</u>

- Calories: 74
- Fat: 0.7g
- Carbohydrates: 16g
- Protein: 2g

Delightful Pesto Pizza

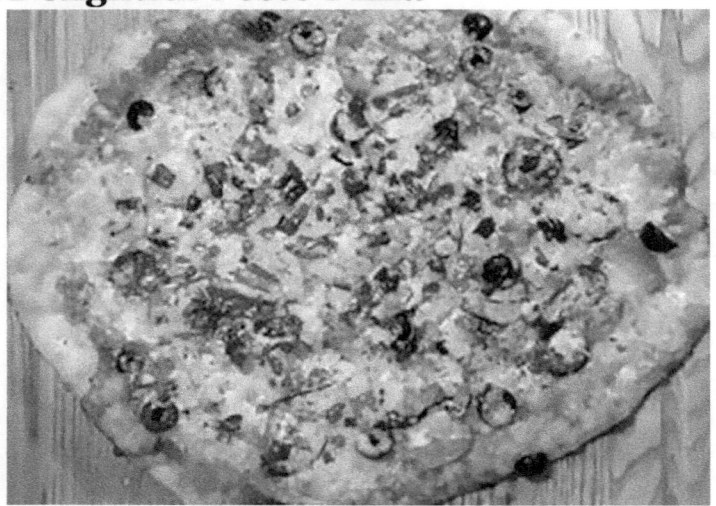

Serving: 4

Prep Time: 25 minutes

Cook Time: 20 minutes

Ingredients

- 1 (10 inch) pizza crust, homemade/premade
- ½ cup sun-dried tomato pesto
- 1 cup button mushrooms, sliced
- 1 red bell pepper, chopped
- 1 cup zucchini, sliced
- 12 cup red onion, thinly sliced
- ½ cup black olives, sliced
- ½ cup Parmesan cheese, grated

How To

1. Pre-heat your oven to 400 degrees Fahrenheit.
2. Line a baking sheet with parchment paper and keep it on the side .

3. Dust the work surface with flour and roll our pizza dough to a 10 inch circle.
4. Transfer dough to baking sheet.
5. Spread pesto over dough (leaving 1 inch from edge).
6. Arrange mushrooms, red bell pepper, zucchini, onion and olives on pizza.
7. Top with cheese.
8. Bake for 20 minutes until golden and crispy.

Nutrition (Per Serving)

- Calories: 210
- Fat: 9g
- Carbohydrates: 25g
- Protein: 9g

Linguine Dredged in Tomato Clam Sauce

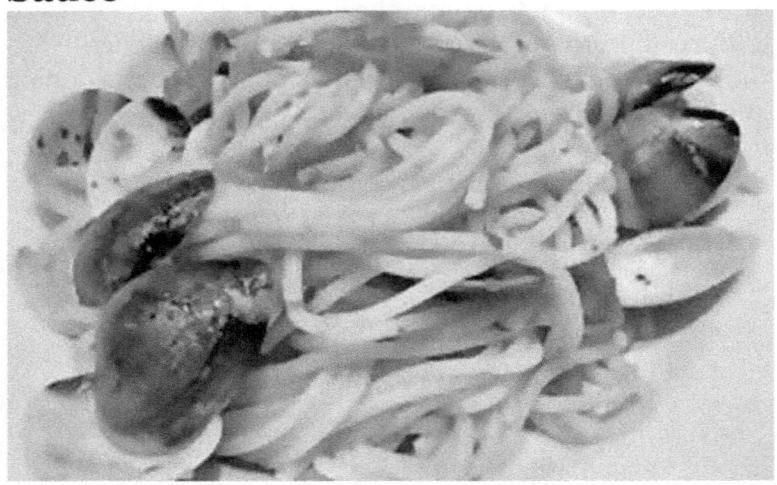

Serving: 4

Prep Time: 10 minutes

Cook Time: 10 minutes

Ingredients

- 1 pound linguine
- Salt and black pepper as needed
- 1 teaspoon extra virgin olive oil
- 1 tablespoon garlic, minced
- 1 teaspoon fresh thyme, chopped
- ½ teaspoon red pepper flakes
- 1 can (15 ounces) sodium-free tomatoes, diced and drained
- 1 can (15 0unce) can whole baby clams, with juice

How To

1. Cook the linguine accordingly.

2. While linguine cooks, heat olive oil in a large skillet over medium heat.
3. Add garlic, thyme, red pepper flakes and sauté for 3 minutes.
4. Stir in tomatoes and clams.
5. Bring sauce to boil and lower heat to low.
6. Simmer for 5 minutes.
7. Season with salt and pepper.
8. Drain cooked pasta and toss with sauce.
9. Garnish with parsley and serve.
10. Enjoy!

<u>Nutrition (Per Serving)</u>

- Calories: 394
- Fat: 5g
- Carbohydrates: 66g
- Protein: 23g

Wild Mushrooms and Pork Chops

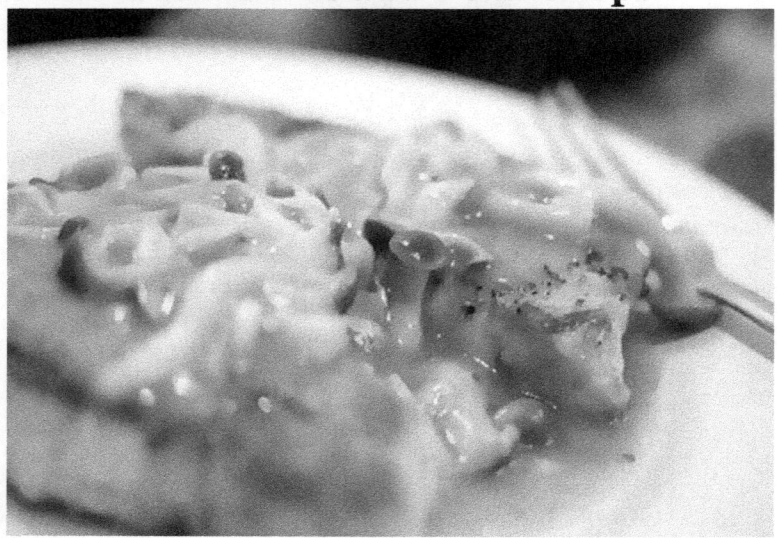

Serving: 4

Prep Time: 10 minutes

Cook Time: 25 minute

Ingredients

- 4 (5 ounce) bone-in-center pork chops
- ¼ teaspoon sea salt
- ¼ teaspoon freshly ground black pepper
- 1 tablespoon extra-virgin olive oil
- 1 sweet onion, chopped
- 2 teaspoons garlic, minced
- 1 pound mixed wild mushrooms, sliced
- 1 teaspoon fresh thyme, chopped
- ½ cup sodium free chicken stock

How To

1. Pat pork chops dry with kitchen towel and season with salt and pepper.

2. Take a large skillet and place it over medium-high heat.
3. Add olive oil and heat it up.
4. Add pork chops and cook for 6 minutes, brown both sides.
5. Transfer meat to platter and keep aside.
6. Add onion and garlic and sauté for 3 minutes.
7. Stir in mushrooms and thyme and sauté for 6 minutes until the mushrooms are caramelized.
8. Return pork chops to the skillet and pour chicken stock.
9. Cover and bring liquid to boil.
10. Reduce heat to low and simmer for 10 minutes.
11. Serve and enjoy!

Nutrition (Per Serving)

- Calories: 308
- Fat: 17g
- Carbohydrates: 7g
- Protein: 33g

Mediterranean Lamb Chops

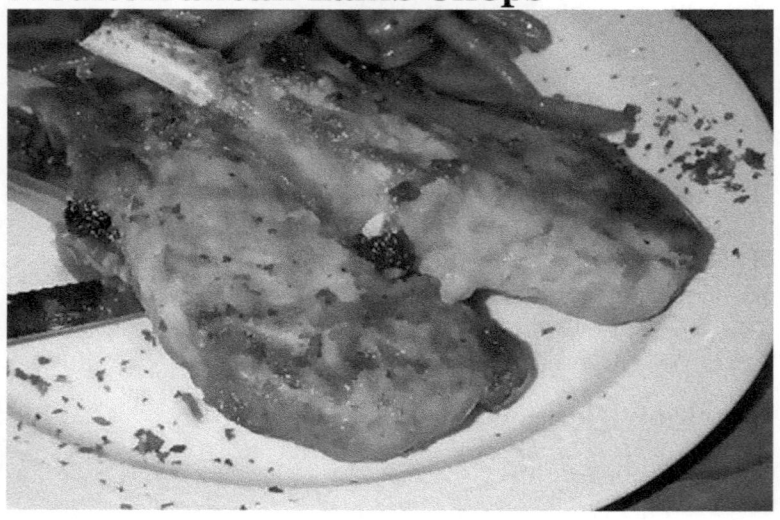

Serving: 4

Prep Time: 10 minutes

Cook Time: 10 minute

Ingredients

- 4 lamb shoulder chops, 8 ounce each
- 2 tablespoons Dijon mustard
- 2 tablespoons Balsamic vinegar
- 1 tablespoon garlic, chopped
- ½ cup olive oil
- 2 tablespoons shredded fresh basil

How To

1. Pat your lamb chop dry using kitchen towel and arrange them on a shallow glass baking dish.
2. Take a bowl and whisk in Dijon mustard, balsamic vinegar, garlic, pepper and mix well.
3. Whisk in the oil very slowly into the marinade until the mixture is smooth.

4. Stir in basil.
5. Pour the marinade over the lamb chops and stir to coat both sides well.
6. Cover the chops and allow them to marinate for 1-4 hours (chilled).
7. Take the chops out and leave them for 30 minutes to allow the temperature to reach normal level.
8. Pre-heat your grill to medium heat and add oil to the grate.
9. Grill the lamb chops for 5-10 minutes per side until both sides are browned.
10. Once the center of the chop reads 145 degree Fahrenheit, the chops are ready, serve and enjoy!

Nutrition (Per Serving)

- Calories: 521
- Fat: 45g
- Carbohydrates: 3.5g
- Protein: 22g

Mushroom and Beef Risotto

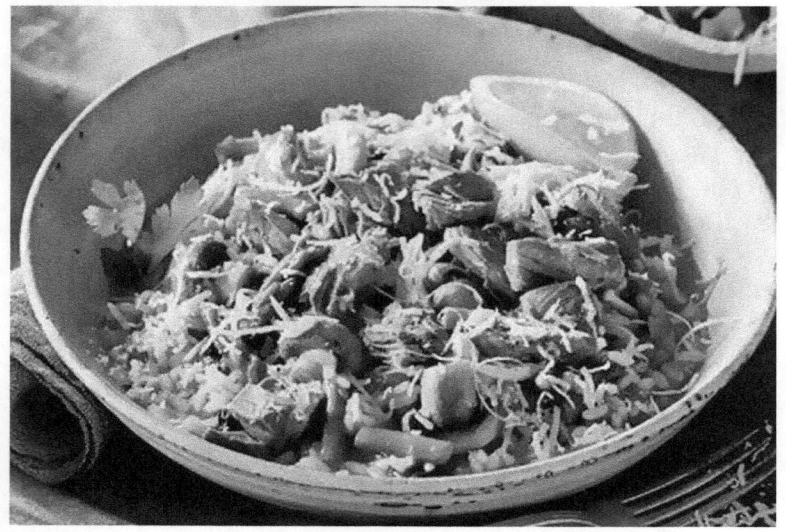

Serving: 4

Prep Time: 5 minutes

Cook Time: 10 minutes

Ingredients

- 2 cups low-sodium beef stock
- 2 cups water
- 2 tablespoon olive oil
- ½ cup scallions, chopped
- 1 cup Arborio rice
- ¼ cup dry white wine
- 1 cup roast beef, thinly stripped
- 1 cup button mushrooms
- ½ cup canned cream of mushroom
- Salt and pepper as needed
- Oregano, chopped
- Parsley, chopped

How To

1. Take a stock pot and put it over medium heat.
2. Add water with beef stock in it.
3. Bring the mixture to a boil and remove the heat.
4. Take another heavy-bottomed saucepan and put it over medium heat.
5. Add in the scallions and stir fry them for 1 minute.
6. Add in the rice then and cook it for at least 2 minutes, occasionally stirring it to ensure that it is finely coated with oil.
7. In the rice mixture, keep adding your beef stock ½ a cup at a time, making sure to stir it often.
8. Once all the stock has been added, cook the rice for another 2 minutes.
9. During the last 5 minutes of your cooking, make sure to add the beef, cream of mushroom, while stirring it nicely.
10. Transfer the whole mix to a serving dish.
11. Garnish with some chopped up parsley and oregano.
12. Serve hot.

Nutrition (Per Serving)

- Calories: 378
- Fat: 12g
- Carbohydrates: 41g
- Protein: 23g

Broiled Mushrooms Burgers and Goat Cheese

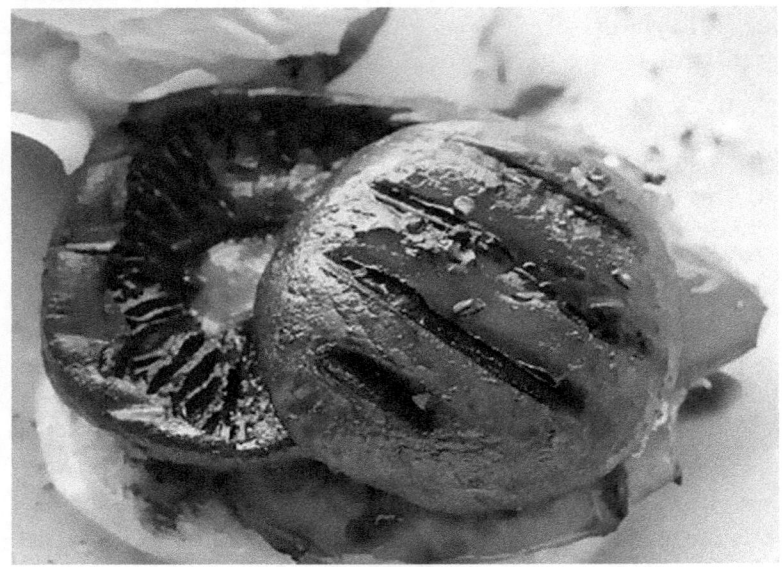

Serving: 4

Prep Time: 15 minutes

Cook Time: 5 minutes

Ingredients

- 4 large Portobello mushroom caps
- 1 red onion, cut into ¼ inch thick slices
- 2 tablespoons extra virgin olive oil
- 2 tablespoons balsamic vinegar
- Pinch of salt
- ¼ cup goat cheese
- ¼ cup sun-dried tomatoes, chopped
- 4 ciabatta buns
- 1 cup kale, shredded

How To

1. Pre-heat your oven to broil.
2. Take a large bowl and add mushrooms caps, onion slices, olive oil, balsamic vinegar and salt.
3. Mix well.
4. Place mushroom caps (bottom side up) and onion slices on your baking sheet.
5. Take a small bowl and stir in goat cheese and sun dried tomatoes.
6. Toast the buns under the broiler for 30 seconds until golden.
7. Spread the goat cheese mix on top of each bun.
8. Place mushroom cap and onion slice on each bun bottom and cover with shredded kale.
9. Put everything together and serve.
10. Enjoy!

<u>Nutrition (Per Serving)</u>

- Calories: 327
- Fat: 11g
- Carbohydrates: 49g
- Protein: 11g

Tuna and Potato Salad

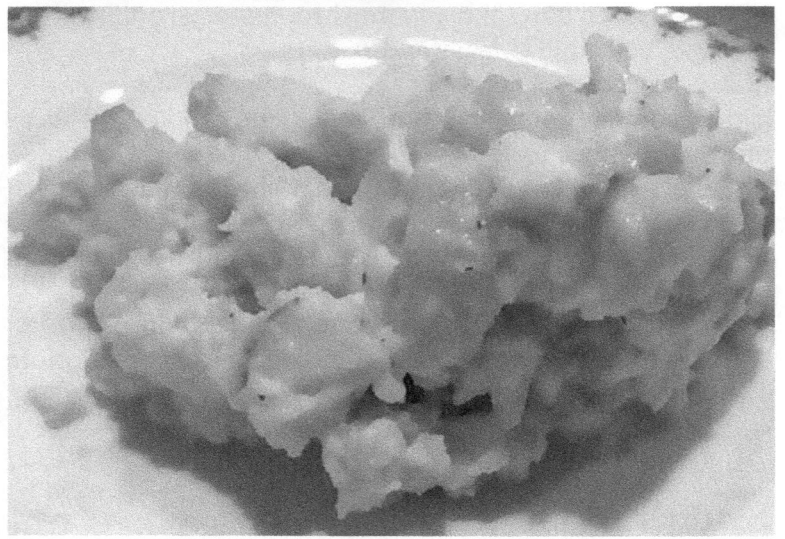

Serving: 4

Prep Time: 10 minutes

Cook Time: nil

Ingredients

- 1 pound baby potatoes, scrubbed, boiled
- 1 cup tuna chunks, drained
- 1 cup cherry tomatoes, halved
- 1 cup medium onion, thinly sliced
- 8 pitted black olives
- 2 medium hard-boiled eggs, sliced
- 1 head Romaine lettuce
- Honey lemon mustard dressing
- ¼ cup olive oil
- 2 tablespoons lemon juice
- 1 tablespoon Dijon mustard
- 1 teaspoon dill weed, chopped
- Salt as needed

- Pepper as needed

How To

1. Take a small glass bowl and mix in your olive oil, honey, lemon juice, Dijon mustard and dill.
2. Season the mix with pepper and salt.
3. Add in the tuna, baby potatoes, cherry tomatoes, red onion, green beans, black olives and toss. everything nicely.
4. Arrange your lettuce leaves on a beautiful serving dish to make the base of your salad.
5. Top them with your salad mixture and place the egg slices.
6. Drizzle it with the previously prepared Salad Dressing.
7. Serve hot.

Nutrition (Per Serving)

- Calories: 406
- Fat: 22g
- Carbohydrates: 28g
- Protein: 26g

Parmesan and Chicken Veggie

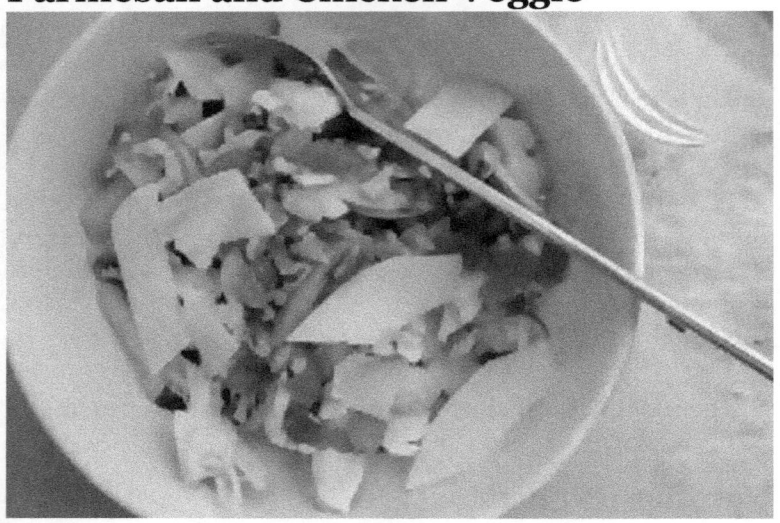

Serving: 4

Prep Time: 5 minutes

Cook Time: 0 minute

Ingredients

- 3 cups cooked shell pasta
- 2 cups baby spinach, torn
- 1 cup roasted cherry tomatoes, halved
- 8 ounces roasted chicken breast, cut into strips
- ¼ cup Parmesan cheese, grated
- Lemon vinaigrette dressing
- 1/3 cup extra-virgin olive oil
- 2 tablespoons lemon juice
- 1 teaspoon lemon zest, finely grated
- ½ teaspoon dried rosemary
- Salt and pepper as needed

How To

1. Take a glass bowl and whisk in oil, zest, lemon juice and rosemary.
2. Keep the mixture to the side.
3. Take another large bowl and add spinach, pasta, cherry tomatoes, chicken and drizzle the dressing on top.
4. Season with salt and pepper.
5. Toss until coated well.
6. Divide the salad amongst serving plates and sprinkle cheese on top.
7. Serve and enjoy!

Nutrition (Per Serving)

- Calories: 398
- Fat: 23g
- Carbohydrates: 24g
- Protein: 24g

Mushroom and Pork Chops

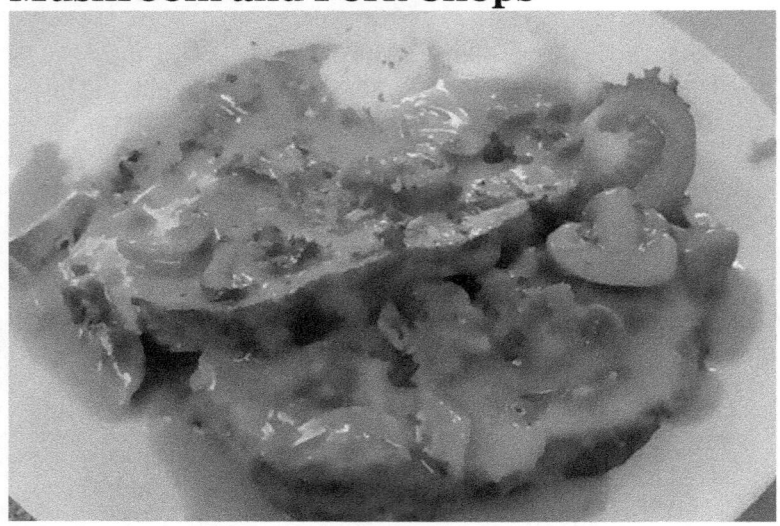

Serving: 4

Prep Time: 10 minutes

Cook Time: 25 minute

Ingredients

- 4 (5 ounce) bone-in-center pork chops
- ¼ teaspoon sea salt
- ¼ teaspoon freshly ground black pepper
- 1 tablespoon extra-virgin olive oil
- 1 sweet onion, chopped
- 2 teaspoons garlic, minced
- 1 pound mixed wild mushrooms, sliced
- 1 teaspoon fresh thyme, chopped
- ½ cup sodium free chicken stock

How To

1. Pat pork chops dry with kitchen towel and season with salt and pepper.

2. Take a large skillet and place it over medium-high heat.
3. Add olive oil and heat it up.
4. Add pork chops and cook for 6 minutes, brown both sides.
5. Transfer meat to platter and keep it aside.
6. Add onion and garlic and sauté for 3 minutes.
7. Stir in mushrooms and thyme and sauté for 6 minutes until the mushrooms are caramelized.
8. Return pork chops to the skillet and pour chicken stock.
9. Cover and bring liquid to boil.
10. Reduce the heat to low and simmer for 10 minutes.
11. Serve and enjoy!

<u>Nutrition (Per Serving)</u>

- Calories: 308
- Fat: 17g
- Carbohydrates: 7g
- Protein: 33g

Oven Roasted Garlic Chicken Thigh

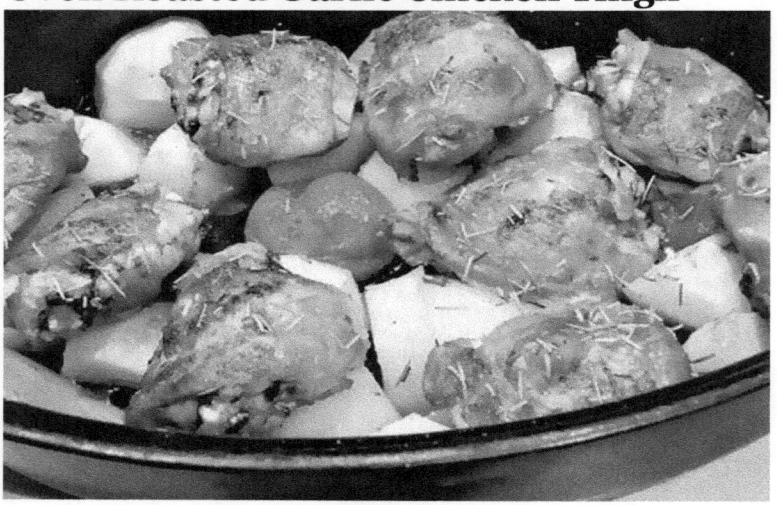

Serving: 4

Prep Time: 10 minutes

Cook Time: 55 minute

Ingredients

- 8 chicken thighs
- Salt and pepper as needed
- 1 tablespoon extra-virgin olive oil
- 6 cloves garlic, peeled and crushed
- 1 jar (10 ounce) roasted red peppers, drained and chopped
- 1 1/2 pounds potatoes, diced
- 2 cups cherry tomatoes, halved
- 1/3 cup capers, sliced
- 1 teaspoon dried Italian seasoning
- 1 tablespoon fresh basil

How To

1. Season chicken with kosher salt and black pepper.

2. Take a cast iron skillet over medium-high heat and heat up olive oil.
3. Sear the chicken on both sides.
4. Add remaining ingredients except basil and stir well.
5. Remove heat and place cast iron skillet in the oven.
6. Bake for 45 minutes at 400 degrees Fahrenheit until the internal temperature reaches 165 degrees Fahrenheit.
7. Serve and enjoy!

Nutrition (Per Serving)

- Calories: 500
- Fat: 23g
- Carbohydrates: 37g
- Protein: 35g

Trout with Wilted Greens

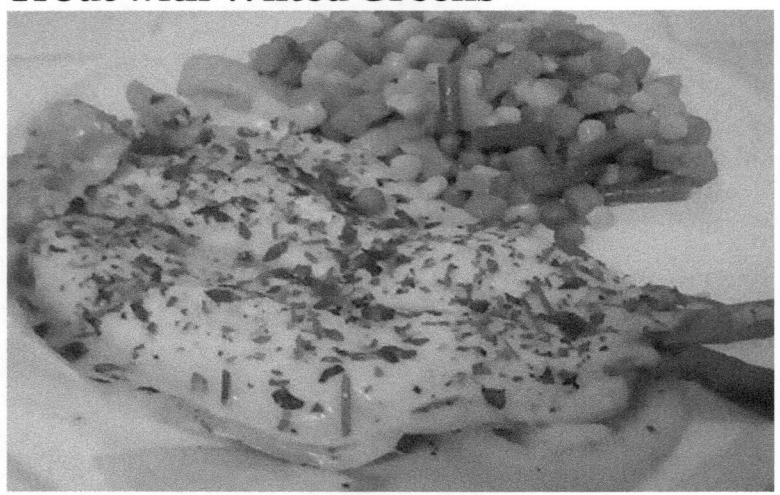

Serving: 4

Prep Time: 5 minutes

Cook Time: 15 minutes

Ingredients

- 2 teaspoons extra virgin olive oil
- 2 cups kale, chopped
- 2 cups Swiss chard, chopped
- ½ sweet onion, thinly sliced
- 4 (5 ounce) boneless skin-on trout fillets
- Juice of 1 lemon
- Sea salt
- Freshly ground pepper
- Zest of 1 lemon

How To

1. Pre-heat your oven to 375 degrees Fahrenheit.
2. Lightly grease a 9 by 13 inch baking dish with olive oil.
3. Arrange the kale, Swiss chard, onion in a dish.

4. Top greens with fish, skin side up and drizzle with olive oil and lemon juice.
5. Season fish with salt and pepper.
6. Bake for 15 minutes until fish flakes.
7. Sprinkle zest.
8. Serve and enjoy!

<u>Nutrition (Per Serving)</u>

- Calories: 315
- Fat: 14g
- Carbohydrates: 6g
- Protein: 39g

Chapter 7: Dinner
Simple Dinnertime Radish and Beet Salad

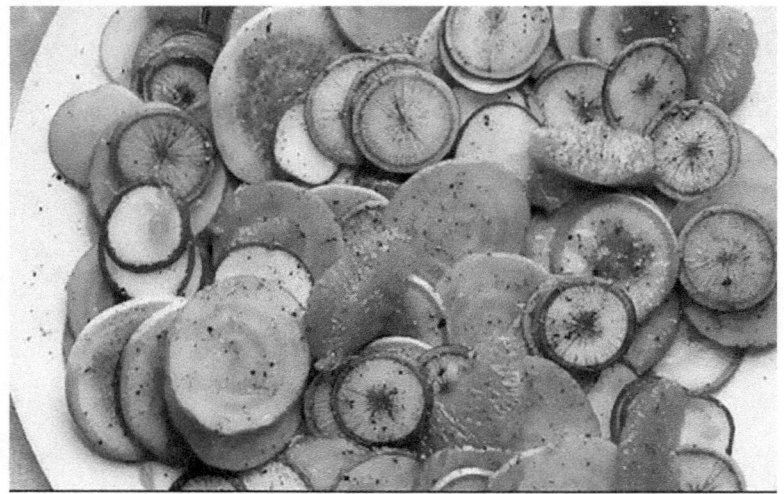

Serving: 4

Prep Time: 15 minutes

Cook Time: 25 minutes

Ingredients

- 10 medium beets, peeled and cut into 1 inch chunks
- 1 teaspoon extra virgin olive oil
- 4 cups seedless watermelon, diced
- 5 large radishes, quartered
- 1 cup kale, shredded
- 1 tablespoon fresh thyme, chopped
- 1 lemon juice
- Sea salt
- Freshly ground black pepper

How To

1. Pre-heat your oven to 350 degrees Fahrenheit.
2. Take a small bowl and add beets, olive oil and toss well to coat the beets.
3. Roast beets for 25 minutes until tender.
4. Transfer to large bowl and cool them.
5. Add watermelon, kale, radish, thyme, lemon juice and toss.
6. Season sea salt and pepper.
7. Serve and enjoy!

Nutrition (Per Serving)

- Calories: 178
- Fat: 2g
- Carbohydrates: 39g
- Protein: 6g

Chicken and Artichoke Salad

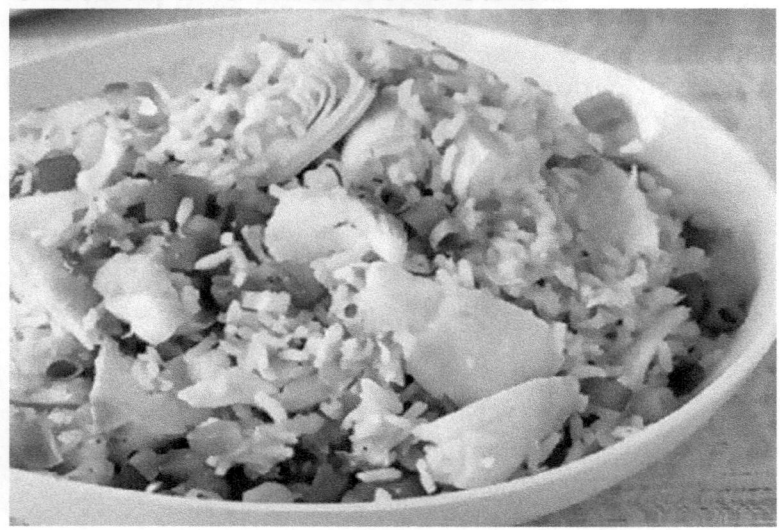

Serving: 4

Prep Time: 10 minutes

Cook Time: 5 minutes

Ingredients

- 2 medium chicken breasts, cooked and cut into 1 inch cubes
- ¼ cup extra virgin olive oil
- 2 cups artichoke hearts, drained and roughly chopped
- 3 large zucchini, diced/cut into small rounds
- 1 can (15 ounce) chickpeas
- 1 cup Kalamata olives
- ½ teaspoon Fresh ground black pepper
- ½ teaspoon Italian seasoning
- ¼ cup Parmesan, grated

How To

1. Take a large skillet and place it over medium heat, heat up olive oil.
2. Add zucchini and Sauté for 5 minutes, season with salt and pepper.
3. Remove from heat and add all the listed ingredients to the skillet.
4. Stir until combined.
5. Transfer to glass container and store.
6. Serve and enjoy!

Nutrition (Per Serving)

- Calories: 457
- Fat: 22g
- Carbohydrates: 30g
- Protein: 24g

Kidney Beans and Cilantro Meal

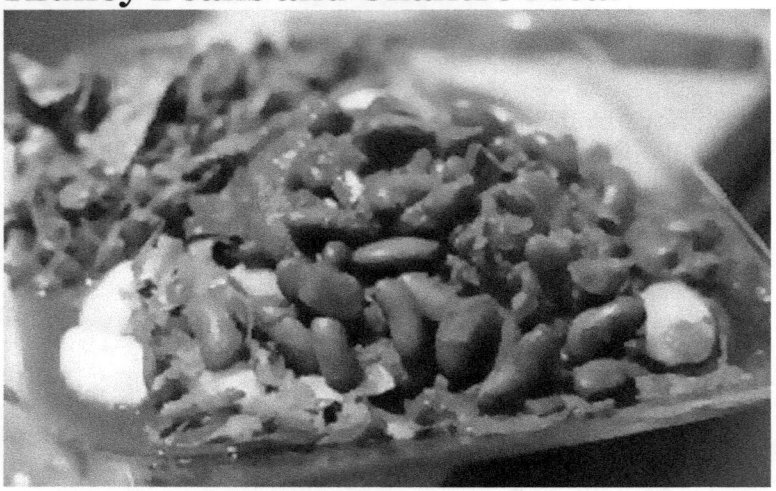

Serving: 6

Prep Time: 5 minutes

Cook Time: nil

Ingredients

- 1 can (15 ounces) kidney beans, drained and rinsed
- ½ English cucumber, chopped
- 1 medium heirloom tomatoes chopped
- 1 bunch fresh cilantro, stems removed and chopped
- 1 red onion, chopped
- Juice of 1 large lime
- 3 tablespoons Dijon mustard
- ½ teaspoon fresh garlic paste
- 1 teaspoon Sumac
- Salt and pepper as needed

How To

1. Take a medium-sized bowl and add kidney beans, chopped up veggies and cilantro.

2. Take a small bowl and make the vinaigrette by adding lime juice, oil, fresh garlic, pepper, mustard and sumac.
3. Pour the vinaigrette over the salad and give it a gentle stir.
4. Add some salt and pepper.
5. Cover it up and allow it to chill for half an hour.
6. Serve!

Nutrition (Per Serving)

- Calories: 74
- Fat: 0.7g
- Carbohydrates: 16g
- Protein: 21g

Caramelized Onion and Fennel Pizza

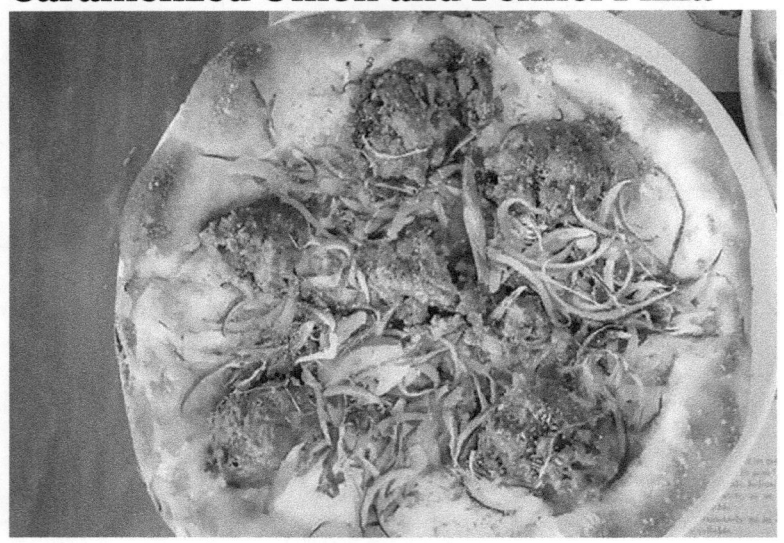

Serving: 4

Prep Time: 15 minutes

Cook Time: 35 minutes

Ingredients

- 1 (10 inch) pizza crust, homemade/premade
- 1 tablespoon extra-virgin olive oil, divided
- 4 cups sweet onion, sliced
- 4 cups fennel, sliced
- 1 teaspoon fresh oregano, chopped
- 1 teaspoon dried thyme
- ¼ teaspoon freshly ground black pepper
- ¼ teaspoon sea salt
- ½ cup Parmesan cheese, grated

How To

1. Pre-heat your oven to 450 degrees Fahrenheit.

2. Place pizza crust on baking sheet and brush edges with 1 tablespoon olive oil.
3. Take a large skillet and place it over medium-high heat.
4. Heat remaining olive oil in the skillet.
5. Add onions, fennel, thyme, oregano, pepper, salt and sauté for 25 minutes.
6. Spread veggies over pizza crust about ½ inch from the edge.
7. Sprinkle vegetables with Parmesan cheese.
8. Bake for 10-12 minutes until crust is crispy.
9. Cut pizza into 8 pieces and serve.
10. Enjoy!

Nutrition (Per Serving)

- Calories: 225
- Fat: 8g
- Carbohydrates: 33g
- Protein: 10g

Lovely Baked Chicken

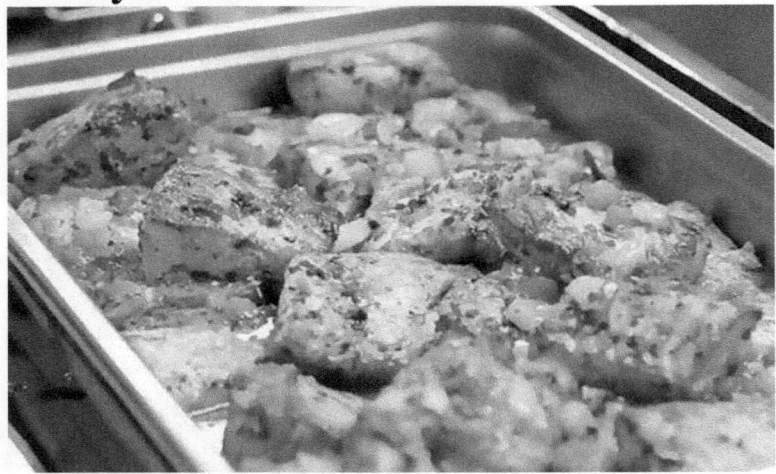

Serving: 2

Prep Time: 10 minutes

Cook Time: 40 minutes

Ingredients

- 2 pieces of 8 ounce skinless and boneless chicken breast
- Salt as needed
- Ground black pepper as needed
- ¼ cup of olive oil
- ¼ cup of freshly squeezed lemon juice
- 1 minced garlic clove
- ½ a teaspoon of dried oregano
- ¼ teaspoon of dried thyme

How To

1. Season breast by rubbing salt and pepper on all sides.
2. Transfer the chicken to a bowl.

3. Take another bowl and add olive oil, oregano, lemon juice, garlic, thyme and mix well.
4. Pour the prepared marinade over the chicken breast and allow it to marinate for 10 minutes.
5. Pre-heat your oven to 400 degrees Fahrenheit.
6. Set the oven rack about 6 inches above the heat source.
7. Transfer the chicken breast to a baking sheet and pour extra marinate on top.
8. Bake for 35-45 minutes until the center is no longer pink.
9. Remove the chicken and place it on the top rack.
10. Broil for 5 minutes more.
11. Enjoy and serve!

Nutrition(Per Serving)

- Calories: 501
- Fat: 32g
- Carbohydrates: 3.5g
- Protein: 47g

Herbed and Lamb Cutlets

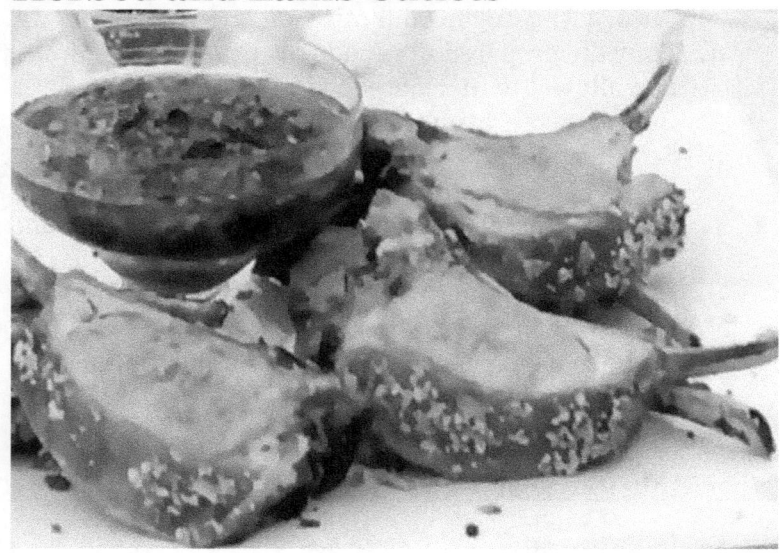

Serving: 6

Prep Time: 15 minutes

Cook Time: 45 minute

Ingredients

- 2 peppers, deseeded and cut into chunky pieces
- 1 large sweet potato, peeled and cut into chunky pieces
- 2 zucchini, sliced into chunks
- 1 red onion, cut in wedges
- 1 tablespoon olive oil
- 8 lean lamb cutlets
- 1 tablespoon thyme leaf, chopped
- 2 tablespoon mint leaves, chopped

How To

1. Pre-heat your oven to a temperature of 392 degrees Fahrenheit.

2. Take a large-sized baking dish and add peppers, zucchini, sweet potatoes and onion.
3. Drizzle oil all over.
4. Season with some ground pepper.
5. Roast for about 25 minutes.
6. Trim off any fat from lamb cutlets (if present).
7. Mix in herbs with a few twists of ground black pepper and pat all over.
8. Take the veggies out of the oven and move them to one side of your tray using a spatula.
9. Place your lamb cutlets on one side and roast for another 10 minutes.
10. Turn the cutlets over and cook for another 10 minutes until the veggies are ready (lightly charred and tender).
11. Mix everything on the tray and enjoy!

Nutrition (Per Serving)

- Calories: 429
- Fat: 29g
- Carbohydrates: 23g
- Protein: 19g

Sweet Potato Curry

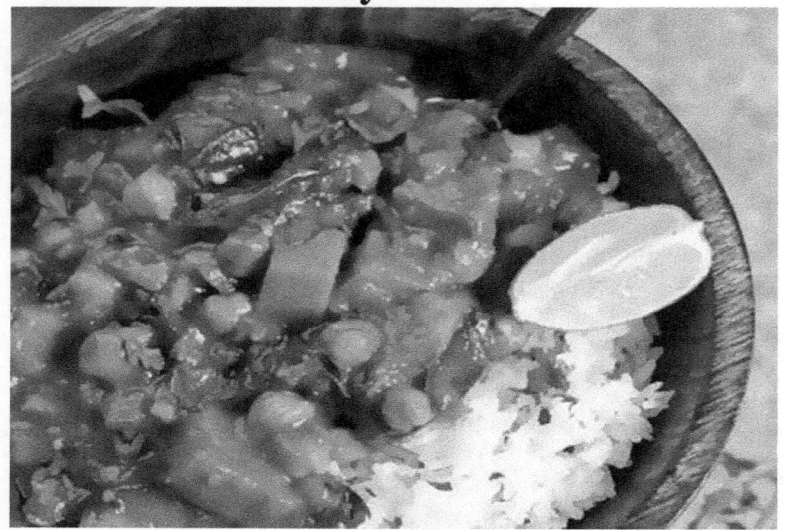

Serving: 4

Prep Time: 15 minutes

Cook Time: 25 minutes

Ingredients

- 1 teaspoon extra virgin olive oil
- 1 sweet onion, peeled and chopped
- 2 teaspoon garlic, minced
- 2 teaspoon ginger, peeled and grated
- 1 cup sodium free vegetable stock
- 3 sweet potatoes, peeled and diced
- 1 large carrot, peeled and diced
- 1 tablespoon curry powder
- 1 teaspoon ground cumin
- ½ teaspoon ground coriander
- ½ teaspoon turmeric
- 1 zucchini, diced
- 1 yellow squash, diced

- 1 red bell pepper, thinly sliced
- ¼ cup water
- 1 tablespoon cornstarch

How To

1. Take a large saucepan and place it over medium-high heat.
2. Add olive oil and heat it up.
3. Add onion, ginger and garlic and sauté for 3 minutes.
4. Stir in broth, sweet potatoes, carrot, curry powder, coriander, cumin, turmeric and bring to a boil.
5. Reduce heat to low and simmer for 15 minutes.
6. Add zucchini, squash, red bell pepper and simmer for 5 minutes .
7. Take a small bowl and stir in water and cornstarch until smooth.
8. Adjust seasoning accordingly and serve.
9. Enjoy!

Nutrition (Per Serving)

- Calories: 208
- Fat: 2g
- Carbohydrates: 45g
- Protein: 4g

Herbed Pork Tenderloin

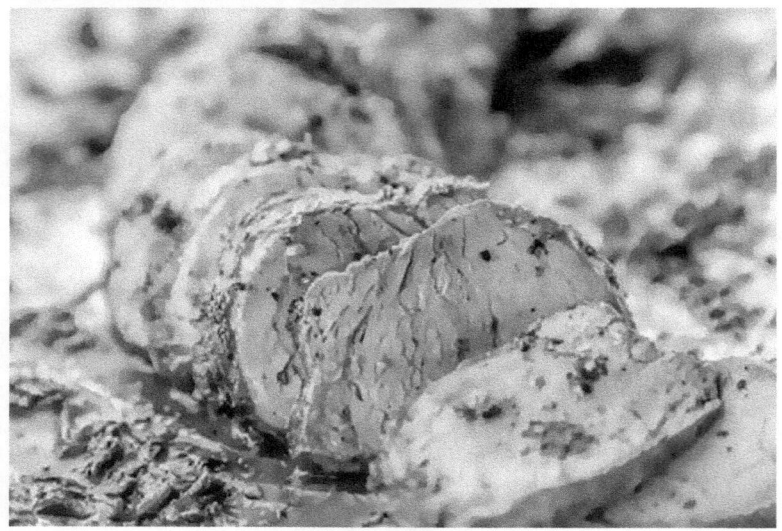

Serving: 8

Prep Time: 10 minutes

Cook Time: 30 minute

Ingredients

- ¼ cup extra virgin olive oil
- ¼ cup fresh oregano, chopped
- 1/ cup parsley, chopped
- 1 tablespoon fresh rosemary, chopped
- 2 teaspoons garlic, minced
- ½ teaspoon red pepper flakes
- ½ teaspoon sea salt
- ½ teaspoon fresh ground black pepper
- 2 pounds pork tenderloin, trimmed of visible fat and silver skin

How To

1. Pre-heat your oven to 400 degrees Fahrenheit.

2. Take a food processor and add ¼ cup olive oil, parsley, oregano, rosemary, garlic, red pepper. flakes, sea salt, pepper and blend until you have a thick paste.
3. Scrape down the sides of the bowl.
4. Rub the herb mix all over the tenderloin.
5. Take a medium ovenproof skillet over medium-high heat.
6. Heat up 1 tablespoon olive oil.
7. Add pork and sear on all sides, turning every 3 minutes until the meat is browned.
8. Place skillet in your oven and roast for 20 minutes until the internal temperature reaches 120-145 degrees Fahrenheit.
9. Remove from oven and let it rest.
10. Slice and serve.
11. Enjoy!

Nutrition (Per Serving)

- Calories: 227
- Fat: 10g
- Carbohydrates: 2g
- Protein: 30g

Green Bean Stew

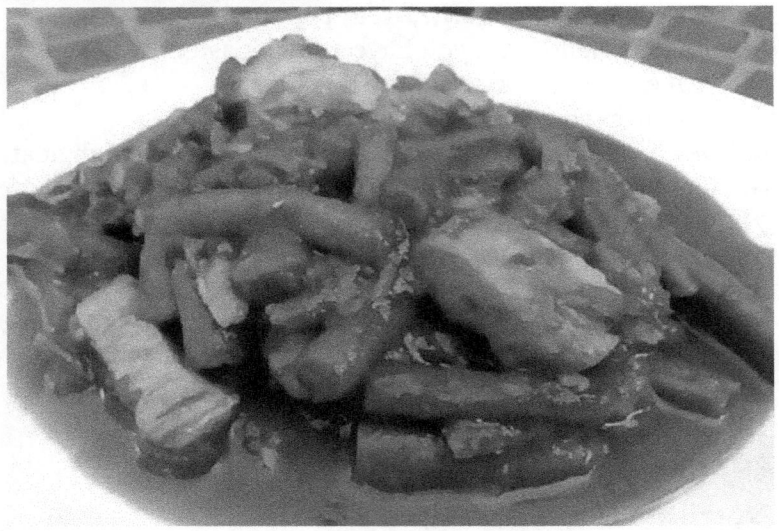

Serving: 4

Prep Time: 10 minutes

Cook Time: 40 minutes

Ingredients

- ¼ cup extra virgin olive oil
- 3 garlic cloves, chopped
- 1 sweet onion, chopped
- Sea salt
- Freshly ground black pepper
- 1 pound fresh green beans, ends snipped and cut into 2 inch pieces
- 1 (8 ounce) can tomato sauce
- ½ cup water

How To

1. Take a small skillet and place over medium heat.
2. Add olive oil and heat it up.

3. Add garlic and onion and sauté for 3 minutes until the garlic is fragrant.
4. Season with salt and pepper.
5. Add beans to the skillet and stir gently with a spoon, cover and cook for 10 minutes.
6. Stir in tomato sauce and water.
7. Cover and cook for 25 minutes more.
8. Serve and enjoy!

Nutrition (Per Serving)

- Calories: 159
- Fat: 13g
- Carbohydrates: 12g
- Protein: 3g

Mediterranean Roast Chicken

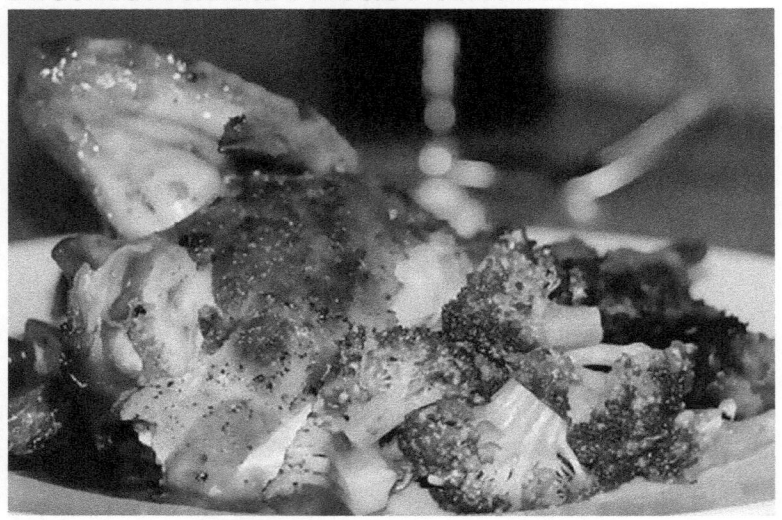

Serving: 6

Prep Time: 60 minutes

Cook Time: 30 minutes

Ingredients

- Juice of 1 large orange
- ¼ cup of Dijon mustard
- ¼ cup of olive oil
- 4 teaspoon of dried Greek oregano
- Salt as needed
- Ground black pepper as needed
- 12 peeled and cubed potatoes
- 5 minced garlic cloves
- 1 whole chicken

How To

1. Pre-heat your oven to 375 degrees Fahrenheit.

2. Take a bowl and whisk in orange juice, Dijon mustard, Greek oregano, salt and pepper, and give it a nice mix.
3. Add potatoes to the bowl and mix to coat them with the mixture.
4. Transfer the potatoes to a large-sized baking dish.
5. Stuff the garlic cloves into the chicken (under the skin).
6. Transfer the chicken to the bowl with the orange and mix well.
7. Transfer the coated chicken to your baking dish and place it on top of the potatoes.
8. Pour any remaining juice on top of the chicken and potato.
9. Bake for 60-90 minutes until the juices run clear.
10. Remove the chicken and cover with aluminum foil, allow to rest for 10 minutes.
11. Slice and serve!

Nutrition(Per Serving)

- Calories: 724
- Fat: 26g
- Carbohydrates: 81g
- Protein: 3g

Honey Chicken

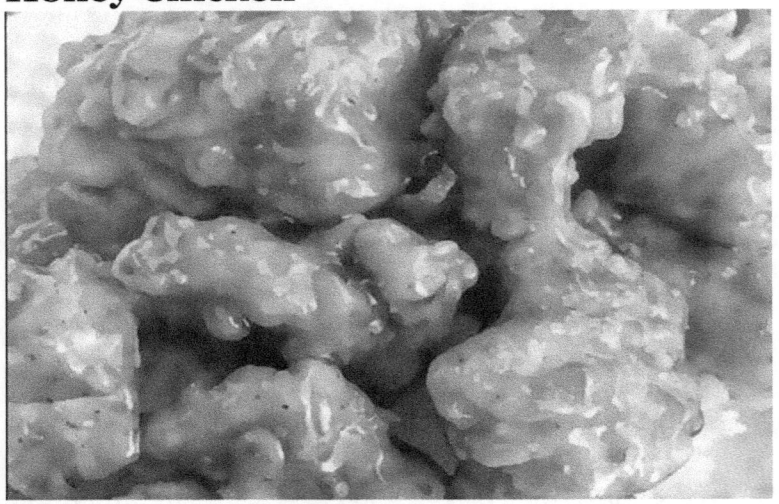

Serving: 4

Prep Time: 10 minutes

Cook Time: 55 minute

Ingredients

- 8 chicken thighs
- Salt and pepper as needed
- 1 tablespoon extra-virgin olive oil
- 6 cloves garlic, peeled and crushed
- 1 jar (10 ounce) roasted red peppers, drained and chopped
- 1 1/2 pounds potatoes, diced
- 2 cups cherry tomatoes, halved
- 1/3 cup capers, sliced
- 1 teaspoon dried Italian seasoning
- 1 tablespoon fresh basil

How To

1. Mix flour, salt and pepper in a bowl and dredge chicken in the seasoned flour.
2. Heat oil in a large skillet and pan fry the chicken for 3-5 minutes per side, making sure to season with pepper.
3. Remove chicken from pan and add asparagus.
4. Sauté until the color brightens and asparagus is tender.
5. Transfer to plate.
6. Add lemon slices and brown them; transfer them to plate as well.
7. Take a bowl and mix lemon zest, honey and 2 tablespoons butter, whisk well.
8. Pour the sauce into a skillet and whisk until the butter melts and the sauce is ready.
9. Serve chicken and asparagus by topping with lemon slices and drizzling butter sauce on top.
10. Enjoy!

Nutrition (Per Serving)

- Calories: 402
- Fat: 21g
- Carbohydrates: 18g
- Protein: 34g

Lovingly Broiled Calamari

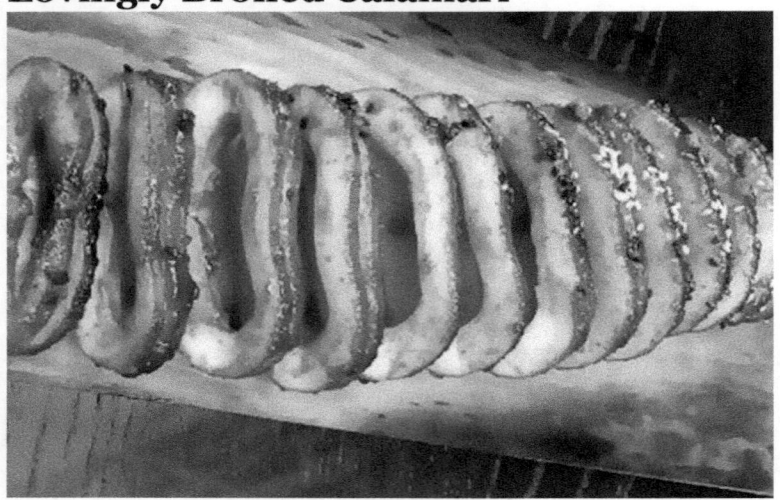

Serving: 4

Prep Time: 10 minutes +1 hour marinating

Cook Time: 8 minutes

Ingredients

- 2 tablespoons extra virgin olive oil
- 1 teaspoon chili powder
- ½ teaspoon ground cumin
- Zest of 1 lime
- Juice of 1 lime
- Dash of sea salt
- 1 ½ pounds squid, cleaned and split open, with tentacles cut into ½ inch rounds
- 2 tablespoons cilantro, chopped
- 2 tablespoons red bell pepper, minced

How To

1. Take a medium bowl and stir in olive oil, chili powder, cumin, lime zest, sea salt, lime juice and pepper.

2. Add squid, stir to coat and let it marinade in the refrigerator for 1 hour.
3. Pre-heat your oven to broil.
4. Arrange squid on a baking sheet, broil for 8 minutes, turning once until tender.
5. Garnish the broiled calamari with cilantro and red bell pepper.
6. Serve and enjoy!

Nutrition (Per Serving)

- Calories: 159
- Fat: 13g
- Carbohydrates: 12g
- Protein: 3g

Broccoli and Tilapia Meal

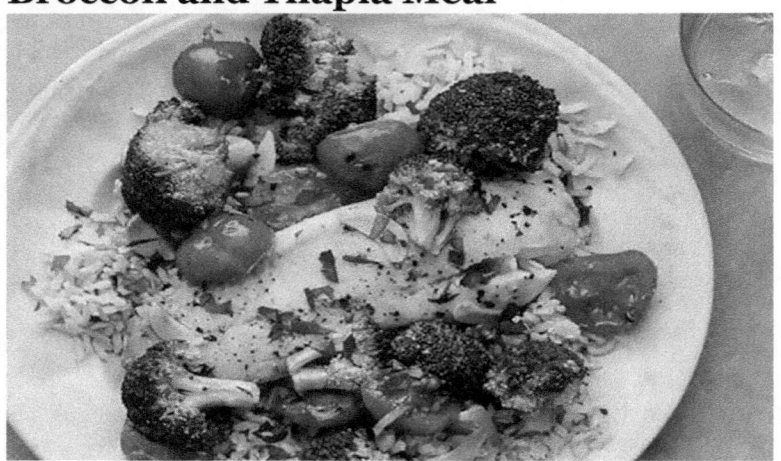

Serving: 4

Prep Time: 4 minutes

Cook Time: 14 minute

Ingredients

- 1 cup broccoli florets, fresh
- 1 tablespoon garlic, minced
- 1 teaspoon lemon pepper seasoning
- 6 ounces tilapia, frozen
- 1 tablespoon butter

How To

1. Pre-heat your oven to 350 degrees Fahrenheit.
2. Add fish in aluminum foil packets.
3. Arrange broccoli around fish.
4. Sprinkle lemon pepper on top.
5. Close the packets and seal.
6. Bake for 14 minutes.
7. Take a bowl and add garlic and butter, mix well and keep the mixture to the side.
8. Remove the packet from the oven and transfer to platter.

9. Place butter on top of the fish and broccoli, serve and enjoy!

Nutrition (Per Serving)

- Calories: 362
- Fat: 25g
- Carbohydrates: 2g
- Protein:29g

Authentic "Medi" Tilapia

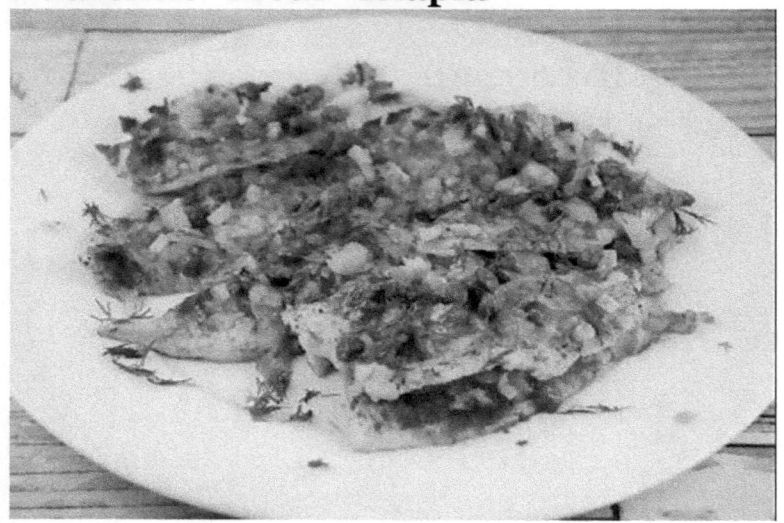

Serving: 4

Prep Time: 15 minutes

Cook Time: 15 minute

Ingredients

- 3 tablespoons sun-dried tomatoes, packed in oil, drained and chopped
- 1 tablespoon capers, drained
- 2 tilapia fillets
- 1 tablespoon oil from sun-dried tomatoes
- 1 tablespoon lemon juice
- 2 tablespoons Kalamata olives, chopped and pitted

How To

10. Pre-heat your oven to 372 degrees Fahrenheit.
11. Take a small-sized bowl and add sun-dried tomatoes, olives, capers and stir well.
12. Keep the mixture to the side.

13. Take a baking sheet and transfer the tilapia fillets and arrange them side by side.
14. Drizzle olive oil all over them.
15. Drizzle lemon juice.
16. Bake in your oven for 10-15 minutes.
17. After 10 minutes, check the fish for a "Flaky" texture.
18. Once cooked properly, top the fish with tomato mix and serve!

<u>Nutrition (Per Serving)</u>

- Calories: 183
- Fat: 8g
- Carbohydrates: 18g
- Protein:183g

Premium and Healthy Chicken Cacciatore

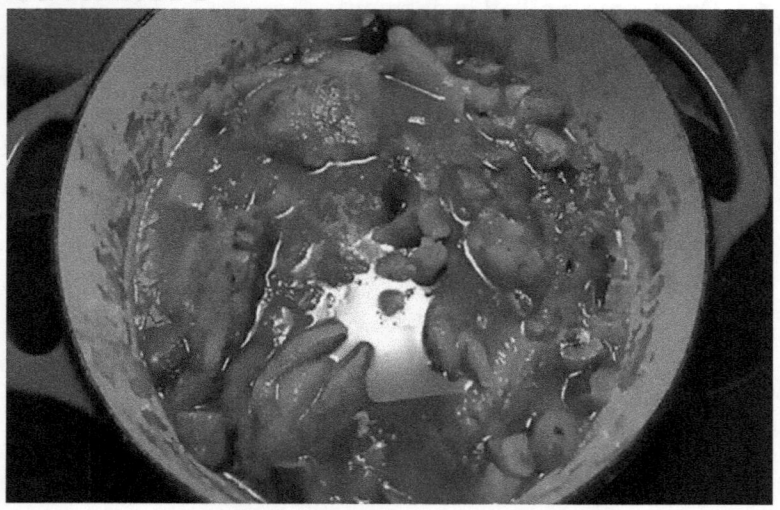

Serving: 8

Prep Time: 5 minutes

Cook Time: 37 minutes

Ingredients

- 2 tablespoon of extra-virgin olive oil
- 1 medium-sized chopped up onion
- 3 tablespoons of chopped up garlic
- 1 whole-sized chicken cut up into 8 pieces
- 1 medium-sized carrot cubed up
- 1 cubed up medium-sized potato
- 1 medium-sized thinly sliced red bell pepper
- 2 cups of stewed tomatoes
- 1 cup of tomato sauce
- ½ cup of green peas
- 1 teaspoon of dried thyme
- Salt as needed
- Ground black pepper as needed

How To

1. Take a large-sized saucepan and place it over medium high heat.
2. Add oil and allow the oil to heat up.
3. Stir in garlic and onion and cook for 2 minutes.
4. Add chicken and cook for 7 minutes.
5. Stir well.
6. Add carrots, red bell pepper, potato, stewed tomatoes, tomato sauce, green peas, thyme and mix.
7. Reduce the heat to low and simmer for 30 minutes.
8. Season with pepper and salt.
9. Transfer to serving dish and enjoy!

Nutrition(Per Serving)

- Calories: 281
- Fat: 8g
- Carbohydrates: 14g
- Protein: 39g

Heavenly Poached Salmon

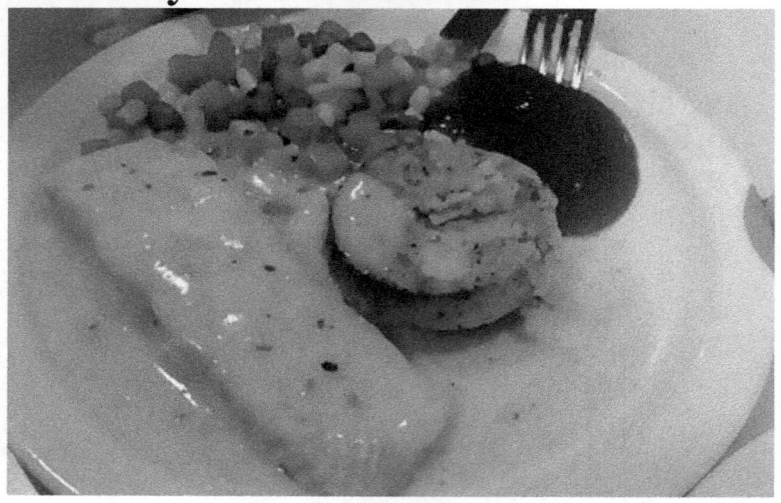

Serving: 4

Prep Time: 10 minutes

Cook Time: 40 minutes

Ingredients

- 6 cups water
- ½ cup freshly squeezed lemon juice
- Juice of 1 lime
- Zest of 1 lime
- 1 sweet onion, thinly sliced
- 1 cup celery leaves, coarsely chopped
- 1 tablespoon fresh dill, chopped
- 1 tablespoon fresh thyme, chopped
- 2 dried bay leaves
- ½ teaspoon black peppercorns
- ½ teaspoon sea salt
- 1 (24 ounce) salmon side, skinned and deboned, cut into 4 pieces

How To

1. Take a large saucepan and place it over medium-high heat.
2. Stir water, lime juice, lemon juice, lime zest, onion, celery, greens, thyme, dill and bay leaves.
3. Strain the liquid through a fine mesh sieve, discard any solids.
4. Pour strained poaching liquid into large skillet over low heat.
5. Bring to a simmer.
6. Add fish and cover skillet, poach for 10 minutes until opaque.
7. Remove salmon from liquid and serve.
8. Enjoy!

Nutrition (Per Serving)

- Calories: 248
- Fat: 11g
- Carbohydrates: 4g
- Protein: 34g

Chapter 8: Side Dishes
Summertime Vegetable Chicken Wraps

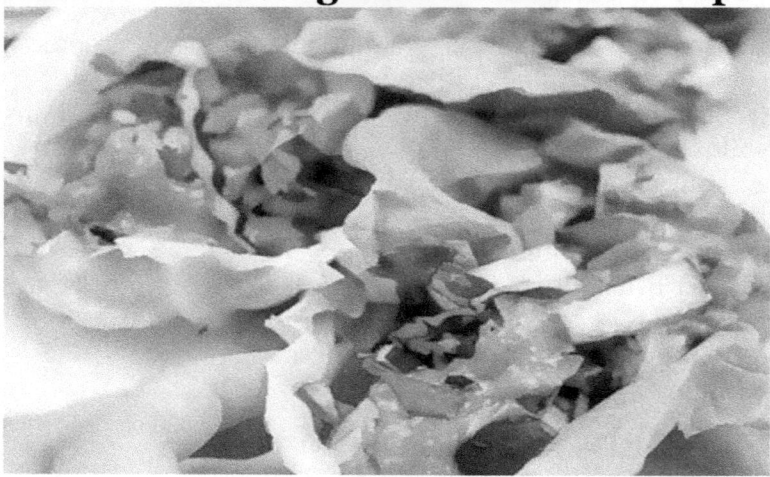

Serving: 4

Prep Time: 15 minutes

Cook Time: nil

Ingredients

- 2 cups cooked chicken, chopped
- ½ English cucumbers, diced
- ½ red bell pepper, diced
- ½ cup carrot, shredded
- 1 scallion, white and green parts, chopped
- ¼ cup plain Greek yogurt
- 1 tablespoon freshly squeezed lemon juice
- ½ teaspoon fresh thyme, chopped
- Pinch of salt
- Pinch of ground black pepper
- 4 multigrain tortillas

How To

1. Take a medium bowl and mix in chicken, red bell pepper, cucumber, carrot, yogurt, scallion, lemon juice, thyme, sea salt and pepper.
2. Mix well.
3. Spoon one quarter of chicken mix into the middle of the tortilla and fold the opposite ends of the tortilla over the filling.
4. Roll the tortilla from the side to create a snug pocket.
5. Repeat with the remaining ingredients and serve.
6. Enjoy!

Nutrition (Per Serving)

- Calories: 278
- Fat: 4g
- Carbohydrates: 28g
- Protein: 27g

Premium Roasted Baby Potatoes

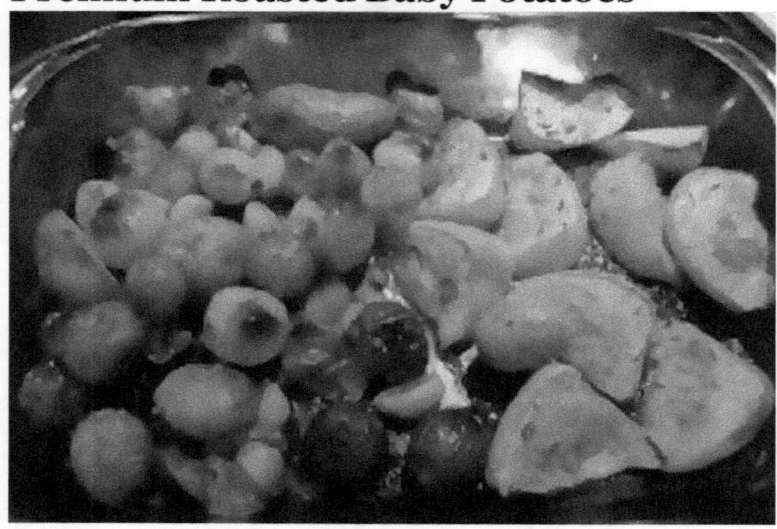

Serving: 4

Prep Time: 10 minutes

Cook Time: 35 minutes

Ingredients

- 2 pounds new yellow potatoes, scrubbed and cut into wedges
- 2 tablespoons extra virgin olive oil
- 2 teaspoons fresh rosemary, chopped
- 1 teaspoon garlic powder
- 1 teaspoon sweet paprika
- ½ teaspoon sea salt
- ½ teaspoon freshly ground black pepper

How To

1. Pre-heat your oven to 400 degrees Fahrenheit.
2. Line baking sheet with aluminum foil and set it aside.

3. Take a large bowl and add potatoes, olive oil, garlic, rosemary, paprika, sea salt and pepper.
4. Spread potatoes in single layer on baking sheet and bake for 35 minutes.
5. Serve and enjoy!

Nutrition (Per Serving)

- Calories: 225
- Fat: 7g
- Carbohydrates: 37g
- Protein: 5g

Tomato and Cherry Linguine

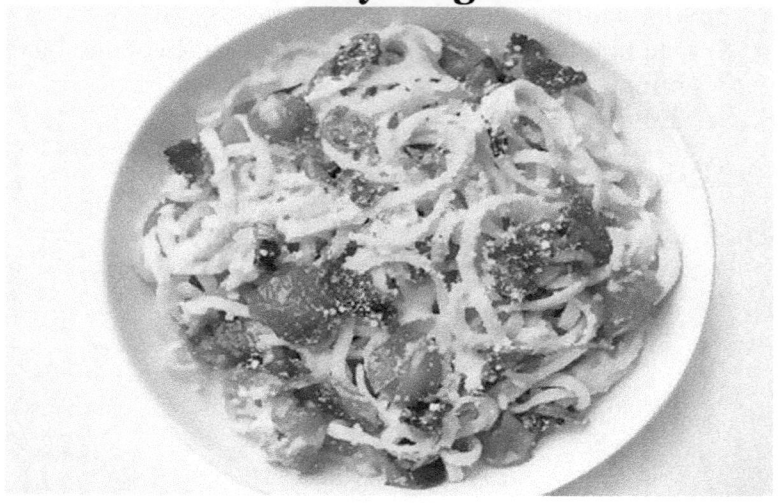

Serving: 4

Prep Time: 10 minutes

Cook Time: 15 minutes

Ingredients

- 2 pounds cherry tomatoes
- 3 tablespoons extra virgin olive oil
- 2 tablespoons balsamic vinegar
- 2 teaspoons garlic, minced
- Pinch of fresh ground black pepper
- ¾ pound whole-wheat linguine pasta
- 1 tablespoon fresh oregano, chopped
- ¼ cup feta cheese, crumbled

How To

1. Pre-heat your oven to 350 degrees Fahrenheit.
2. Line baking sheet with parchment paper and keep aside.
3. Take a large bowl and add cherry tomatoes, 2 tablespoons olive oil, balsamic vinegar, garlic, pepper and toss.

4. Spread tomatoes evenly on baking sheet and roast for 15 minutes.
5. While the tomatoes are roasting, cook the pasta according to the package instructions and drain the paste into a large bowl.
6. Toss pasta with 1 tablespoon olive oil.
7. Add roasted tomatoes (with juice) and toss.
8. Serve with topping of oregano and feta cheese.
9. Enjoy!

Nutrition (Per Serving)

- Calories: 397
- Fat: 15g
- Carbohydrates: 55g
- Protein: 13g

Mediterranean Zucchini Mushroom Pasta

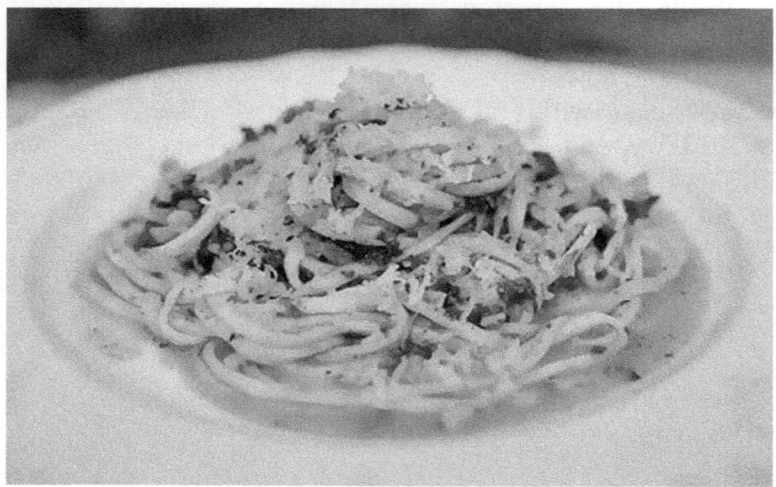

Serving: 4

Prep Time: 10 minutes

Cook Time: 10 minutes

Ingredients

- ½ pound pasta
- 2 tablespoons olive oil
- 6 garlic cloves, crushed
- 1 teaspoon red chili
- 2 spring onions, sliced
- 3 teaspoons rosemary, chopped
- 1 large zucchini, cut in half lengthwise and sliced
- 5 large portabella mushrooms
- 1 can tomatoes
- 4 tablespoons Parmesan cheese
- Fresh ground black pepper

How To

1. Cook the pasta in boiling water until Al Dente.
2. Take a large-sized frying pan and place it over medium heat.
3. Add oil and allow the oil to heat up.
4. Add garlic, onion and chili and sauté for a few minutes until golden.
5. Add zucchini, rosemary and mushroom and sauté for a few minutes.
6. Increase the heat to medium-high and add tinned tomatoes to the sauce until thick.
7. Drain your boiled pasta and transfer to serving platter.
8. Pour the tomato mix on top and mix using tongs.
9. Garnish with Parmesan and freshly ground black pepper.
10. Enjoy!

Nutrition (Per Serving)

- Calories: 361
- Fat: 12g
- Carbohydrates: 47g
- Protein: 14g

Lemon and Garlic Fettucine

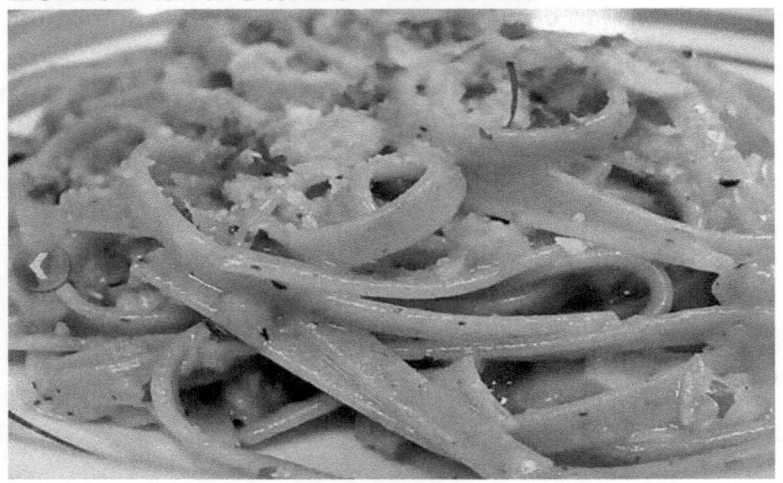

Serving: 5

Prep Time: 5 minutes

Cook Time: 15 minutes

Ingredients

- 8 ounces of whole wheat fettuccine
- 4 tablespoons of extra virgin olive oil
- 4 cloves of minced garlic
- 1 cup of fresh breadcrumbs
- ¼ cup of lemon juice
- 1 teaspoon of freshly ground pepper
- ½ teaspoon of salt
- 2 cans of 4 ounce boneless and skinless sardines (dipped in tomato sauce)
- ½ cup of chopped up fresh parsley
- ¼ cup of finely shredded Parmesan cheese

How To

1. Take a large-sized pot and bring water to a boil.

2. Cook pasta for 10 minutes until Al Dente.
3. Take a small-sized skillet and place it over medium heat.
4. Add 2 tablespoons of oil and allow it to heat up.
5. Add garlic and cook for 20 seconds.
6. Transfer the garlic to a medium-sized bowl
7. Add breadcrumbs to the hot skillet and cook for 5-6 minutes until golden
8. Whisk in lemon juice, pepper and salt into the garlic bowl
9. Add pasta to the bowl (with garlic) and sardines, parsley and Parmesan
10. Stir well and sprinkle bread crumbs
11. Enjoy!

Nutrition(Per Serving)

- Calories: 480
- Fat: 21g
- Carbohydrates: 53g
- Protein: 23g

Roasted Broccoli with Parmesan

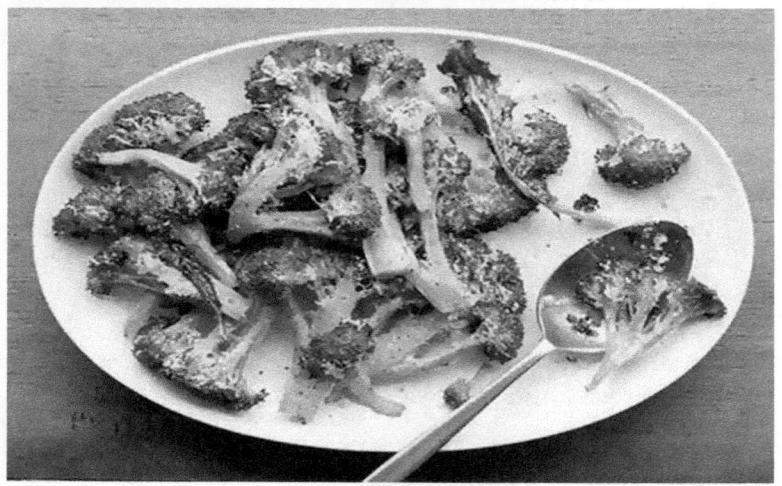

Serving: 4

Prep Time: 10 minutes

Cook Time: 10 minutes

Ingredients

- 2 head broccoli, cut into florets
- 2 tablespoons extra-virgin olive oil
- 2 teaspoons garlic, minced
- Zest of 1 lemon
- Pinch of salt
- ½ cup Parmesan cheese, grated

How To

1. Pre-heat your oven to 400 degrees Fahrenheit.
2. Lightly grease the baking sheet with olive oil and keep it aside.
3. Take a large bowl and add broccoli with 2 tablespoons olive oil, lemon zest, garlic, lemon juice and salt.
4. Spread mix on the baking sheet in single layer and sprinkle with Parmesan cheese.

5. Bake for 10 minutes until tender.
6. Transfer broccoli to serving the dish.
7. Serve and enjoy!

Nutrition (Per Serving)

- Calories: 154
- Fat: 11g
- Carbohydrates: 10g
- Protein: 9g

Spinach and Feta Bread

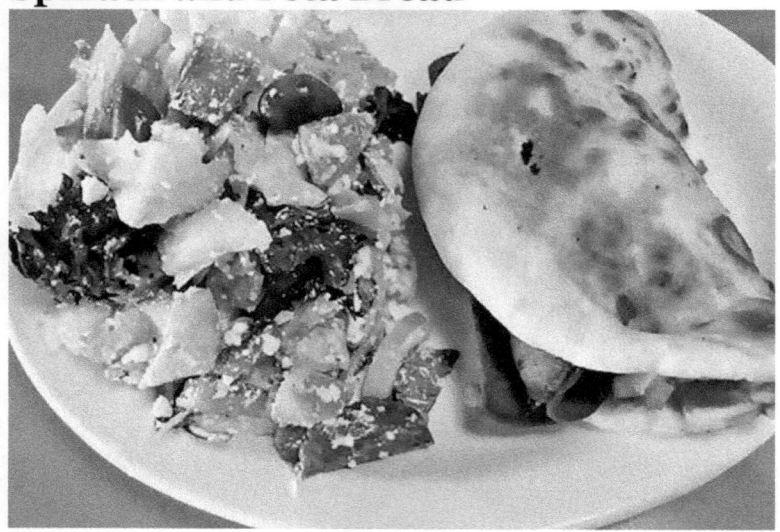

Serving: 6

Prep Time: 10 minutes

Cook Time: 12 minute

Ingredients

- 6 ounces of sun dried tomato pesto
- 6 pieces of 6 inch whole wheat pita bread
- 2 chopped up Roma plum tomatoes
- 1 bunch of rinsed and chopped spinach
- 4 sliced fresh mushrooms
- ½ cup of crumbled feta cheese
- 2 tablespoons of grated Parmesan cheese
- 3 tablespoons of olive oil
- Ground black pepper as needed

How To

1. Pre-heat your oven to a temperature of 350 degrees Fahrenheit.

2. Spread your tomato pesto onto one side of your pita bread and place on your baking sheet (with the pesto side up).
3. Top up the pitas with spinach, tomatoes, feta cheese, mushrooms and Parmesan cheese.
4. Drizzle with some olive oil and season nicely with pepper.
5. Bake in your oven for about 12 minutes until the breads are crispy.
6. Cut up the pita into quarters and serve!

Nutrition(Per Serving)

- Calories: 350
- Fat: 17g
- Carbohydrates: 41g
- Protein:11g

Quick Zucchini Bowl

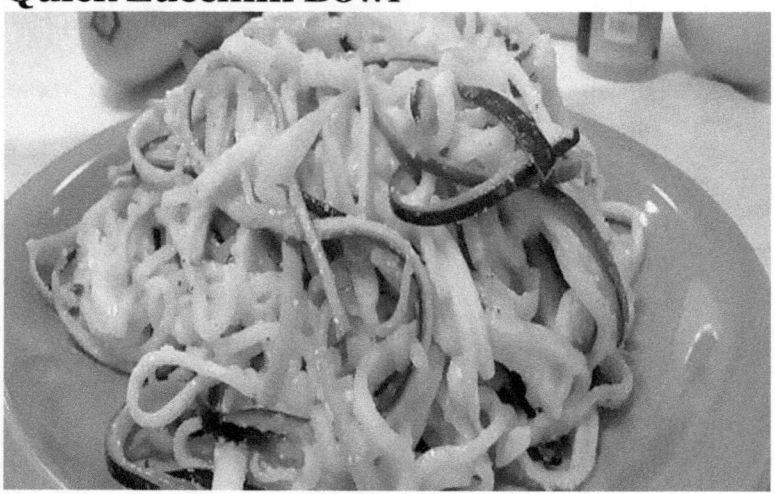

Serving: 4

Prep Time: 10 minutes

Cook Time: 10 minutes

Ingredients

- ½ pound of pasta
- 2 tablespoons of olive oil
- 6 crushed garlic cloves
- 1 teaspoon of red chili
- 2 finely sliced spring onions
- 3 teaspoons of chopped rosemary
- 1 large zucchini cut up in half, lengthways and sliced
- 5 large portabella mushrooms
- 1 can of tomatoes
- 4 tablespoons of Parmesan cheese
- Fresh ground black pepper

How To

1. Cook the pasta in boiling water until Al Dente.

2. Take a large-sized frying pan and place over medium heat.
3. Add oil and allow the oil to heat up.
4. Add garlic, onion and chili and sauté for a few minutes until golden.
5. Add zucchini, rosemary and mushroom and sauté for a few minutes.
6. Increase the heat to medium-high and add tinned tomatoes to the sauce until thick.
7. Drain your boiled pasta and transfer to a serving platter.
8. Pour the tomato mix on top and mix using tongs.
9. Garnish with Parmesan cheese and freshly ground black pepper.
10. Enjoy!

Nutrition(Per Serving)

- Calories: 361
- Fat: 12g
- Carbohydrates: 47g
- Protein: 14g

Healthy Basil Platter

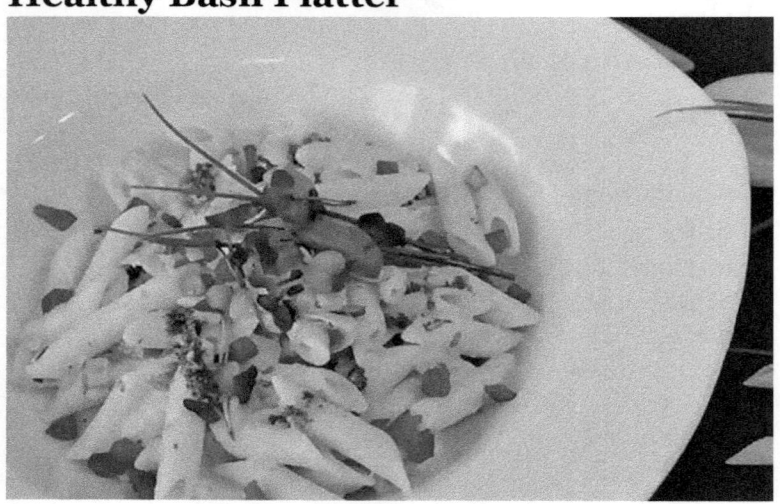

Serving: 4

Prep Time: 25 minutes

Cook Time: 15 minutes

Ingredients

- 2 pieces of red pepper seeded and cut up into chunks
- 2 pieces of red onion cut up into wedges
- 2 mild red chilies, diced and seeded
- 3 coarsely chopped garlic cloves
- 1 teaspoon of golden caster sugar
- 2 tablespoons of olive oil (plus additional for serving)
- 2 pound of small ripe tomatoes quartered up
- 12 ounces of dried pasta
- Just a handful of basil leaves
- 2 tablespoons of grated Parmesan

How To

1. Pre-heat the oven to 392 degrees Fahrenheit.

2. Take a large-sized roasting tin and scatter pepper, red onion, garlic and chilies.
3. Sprinkle sugar on top.
4. Drizzle olive oil and season with pepper and salt.
5. Roast the veggies in your oven for 15 minutes.
6. Take a large-sized pan and cook the pasta in boiling, salted water until Al Dente.
7. Drain them.
8. Remove the veggies from the oven and tip in the pasta into the veggies.
9. Toss well and tear basil leaves on top.
10. Sprinkle Parmesan and enjoy!

Nutrition(Per Serving)

- Calories: 452
- Fat: 8g
- Carbohydrates: 88g
- Protein: 14g

Herbed Up Bruschetta

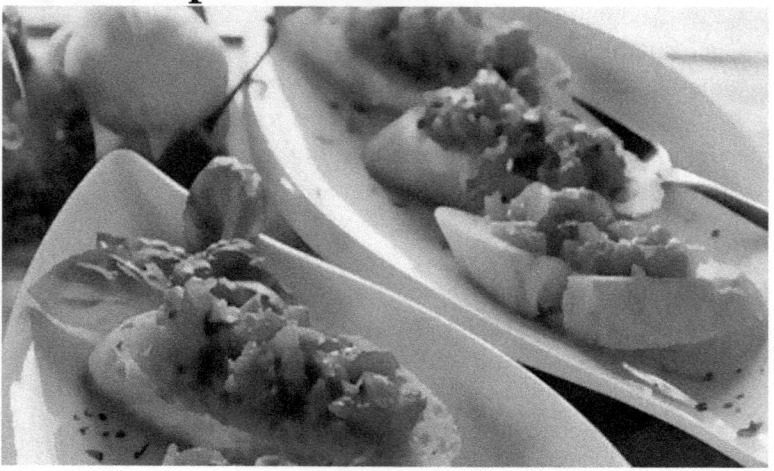

Serving: 12

Prep Time: 12 minutes

Cook Time: 0 minute

Ingredients

- 16 thin slices of toasted French bread
- 2 cups of quartered cherry tomatoes
- 1 finely chopped medium-sized white onion
- Salt as needed
- Ground black pepper as needed
- Fresh sweet basil

For dressing

- ¼ cup of olive oil
- 2 tablespoons of balsamic vinegar
- 1 tablespoon of lemon juice
- 1 tablespoon of Dijon mustard
- 2 tablespoons of minced fresh herbs
- 1 minced clove of garlic

How To

1. Whisk together your olive oil, lemon juice, balsamic vinegar, Dijon mustard, garlic and mixed herbs in a medium-sized bowl.
2. Add the onion and cherry tomatoes.
3. Toss finely to coat it.
4. Season with some pepper and salt.
5. Top each of your bread toast with the previously made tomato mix.
6. Drizzle with some more dressing if you like.
7. Garnish it with fresh basil.
8. Serve.

Nutrition(Per Serving)

- Calories: 118
- Fat: 4g
- Carbohydrates: 18g
- Protein: 4g

Homemade Almond Biscotti

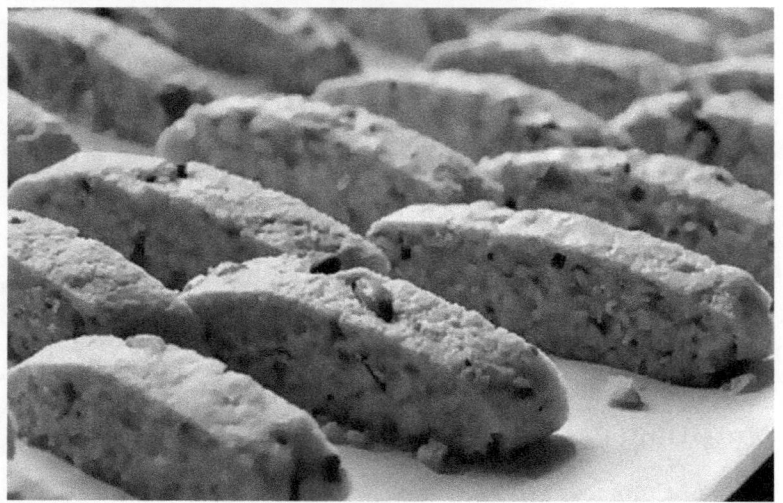

Prep Time: 10 minutes

Cooking Time: 35 minutes

Serving: 30

Ingredients

- 2/3 cups of soft unsalted butter
- ¾ cup and 2 tablespoons of granulated sugar
- 1 teaspoon of crushed anise seed
- 2 whole sized eggs
- 2 tablespoons of amaretto liqueur
- 1 teaspoon of vanilla extract
- 2 ¼ cup of all-purpose flour
- 1 teaspoon of baking powder
- 1 teaspoon of baking soda
- ½ teaspoon of salt
- ¾ cup of chopped up roasted almonds

How To

1. Pre-heat your oven to a temperature of 325 degrees Fahrenheit.
2. Line a cookie sheet with parchment paper.
3. Take an electric mixer and cream your butter.
4. Then, slowly add the sugar and keep mixing until light and fluffy.
5. Add the aniseed.
6. Add the eggs one at a time, making sure to mix after every addition.
7. Stir in your amaretto liqueur alongside the vanilla extract.
8. Slowly add the flour, baking soda and baking powder.
9. Fold in the chopped up almonds.
10. Divide the dough into 2 halves with floured dusted hands and form each of the dough into a rough 12 x 2 and a ½ inch log.
11. Bake your logs for 25 minutes until a fine golden brown texture appears.
12. Cool them on a wire rack.
13. Slice your logs diagonally into ½ inch wide pieces using a serrated knife.
14. Place them in your cookie sheet to make one single layer.
15. Return them to your oven and bake for another 7 minutes until the edges are browned.
16. Serve.

Nutrition

- Calories: 111
- Fat: 6g
- Carbohydrates: 13g
- Protein: 2g

Chapter 9: Dessert
Almond and Chocolate Butter Dip

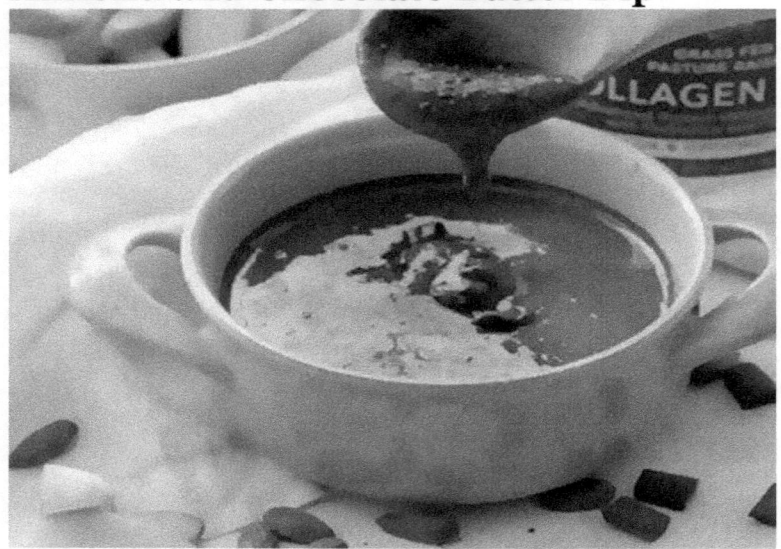

Serving: 14

Prep Time: 15 minutes

Cook Time: 10 minute

Ingredients

- 1 cup Plain Greek Yogurt
- ½ cup almond butter
- 1/3 cup chocolate hazelnut spread
- 1 tablespoon honey
- 1 teaspoon vanilla
- Sliced fruits such as pears, apples, apricots, bananas, etc.

How To

1. Take a medium-sized bowl and add the first five listed ingredients.

2. With an immersion blender, blend well until you have a smooth dip.
3. Serve with your favorite sliced fruit.
4. Enjoy!

Nutrition (Per Serving)

- Calories: 115
- Fat: 8g
- Carbohydrates: 115g
- Protein: 4g

Strawberry and Feta Delight

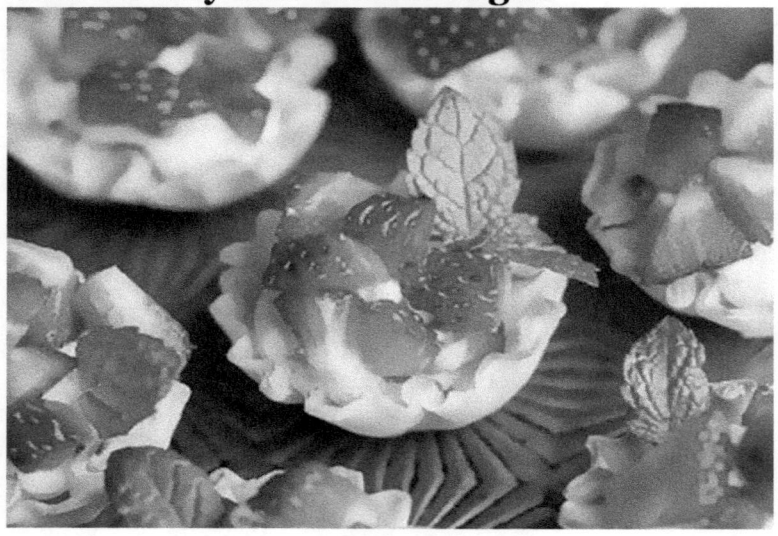

Serving: 4

Prep Time: 10 minutes

Cook Time: nil

Ingredients

- 4 cups baby spinach
- 6 ounces feta cheese, crumbled
- 1 cup fresh strawberries, thinly sliced
- ½ cup walnuts, chopped

Balsamic Dijon vinaigrette

- 2 tablespoons extra-virgin olive oil
- 2 tablespoons balsamic vinegar
- 1 tablespoon Dijon mustard
- 1 tablespoon honey
- Salt and pepper as needed

How To

1. Take a small-sized glass bowl and mix in the olive oil, Dijon mustard, balsamic vinegar and honey.
2. Season with some pepper and salt.
3. Add the spinach, strawberries, feta, walnuts and pine nuts in a large-sized mixing bowl.
4. Divide the mixture amongst serving plates and dress with the previously prepared vinaigrette dressing.
5. Serve

<u>Nutrition (Per Serving)</u>

- Calories: 270
- Fat: 22g
- Carbohydrates: 11g
- Protein: 9g

Simple Strawberry Yogurt Ice Cream

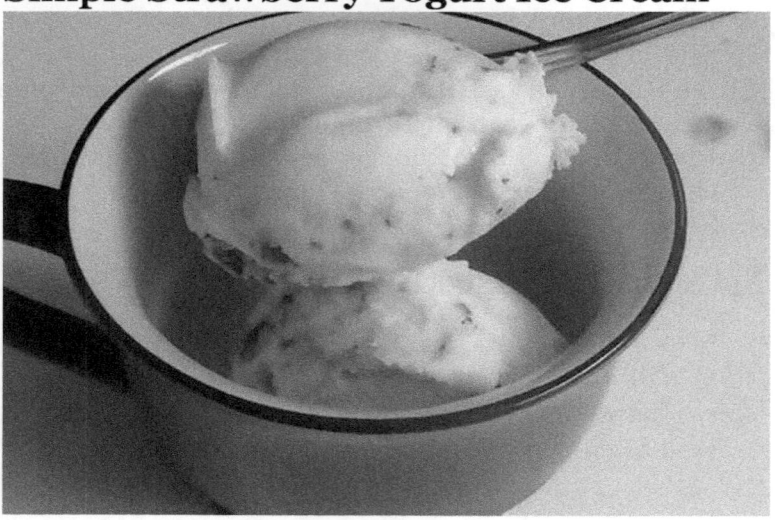

Serving: 4

Prep Time: 10 minutes

Cook Time: 20 minutes

Ingredients

- 3 cups of plain Greek low-fat yogurt
- 1 cup of sugar
- ¼ cup of freshly squeeze lemon juice
- 2 teaspoons of vanilla
- 1/8 teaspoon of salt
- 1 cup of sliced strawberries

How To

1. Take a medium-sized bowl and add yogurt, lemon juice, sugar, vanilla and salt.
2. Whisk the whole mixture well.
3. Freeze the yogurt mix into a 2 quart ice cream maker according to the given instructions.

4. Make sure to add sliced strawberries during the final minute.
5. Transfer the yogurt to an airtight container.
6. Freeze for another 2-4 hours.
7. Allow to stand for about 5-15 minutes.
8. Serve and enjoy!

<u>Nutrition(Per Serving)</u>

- Calories: 86
- Fat: 1g
- Carbohydrates: 16g
- Protein: 4g

Pear with Honey Drizzles

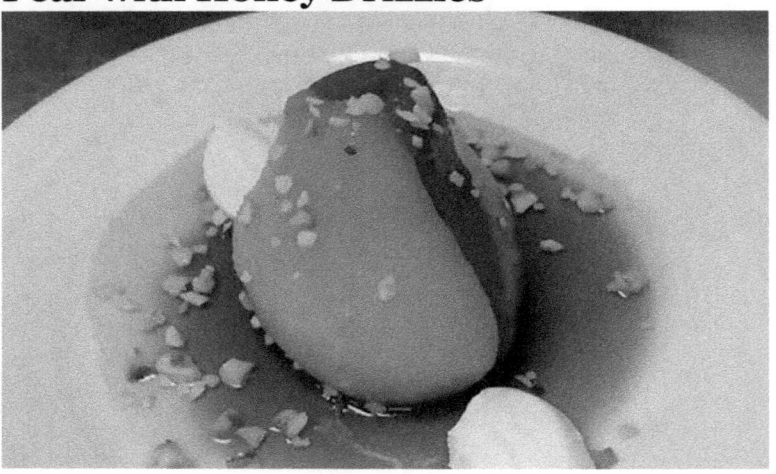

Serving: 4

Prep Time: 10 minutes

Cook Time: 20 minutes

Ingredients

- 3 pieces of ripe medium Bosc of Bartlett pears. Peel and core, then slice into halves
- ¼ cup of pear nectar
- 3 tablespoons of honey
- 2 tablespoons of butter
- 1 teaspoon of orange zest
- ½ cup of mascarpone cheese
- 2 tablespoons of powdered sugar
- 1/3 cup of chopped up roasted salted pistachio

How To

1. Pre-heat your oven to 400 degrees Fahrenheit.
2. Take baking dish and add pears, making sure to arrange them with the cut side facing down.

3. Add the next four listed ingredients.
4. Roast for 20-25 minutes until tender.
5. Transfer the pears to a serving dish and pour the cooking liquid on top.
6. Take a bowl and stir in mascarpone cheese and powdered sugar.
7. Spoon the mix over the pears.
8. Sprinkle with pistachio and drizzle honey.
9. Enjoy!

Nutrition(Per Serving)

- Calories: 250
- Fat: 8g
- Carbohydrates: 27g
- Protein: 3g

Cherry and Olive Bites

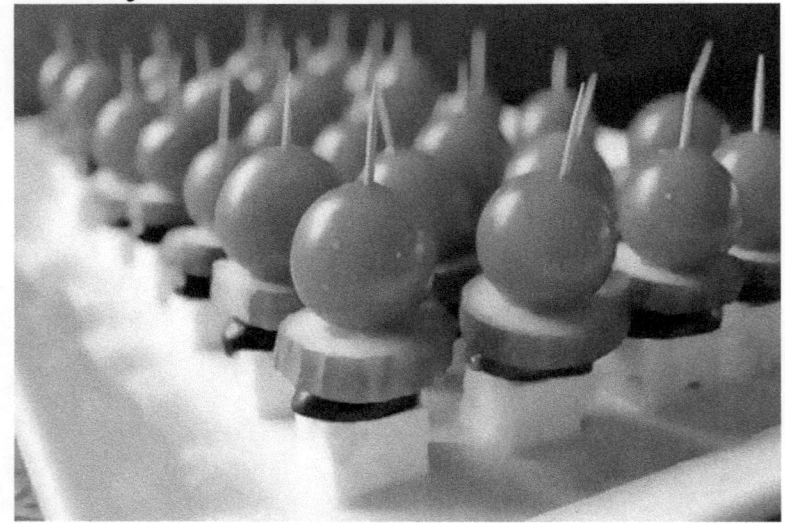

Serving: 30

Prep Time: 15 minutes

Cook Time: nil

Ingredients

- 24 cherry tomatoes, halved
- 24 black olives, pitted
- 24 feta cheese cubes
- 24 toothpick/decorative skewers

How To

1. Use a toothpick or skewer and thread feta cheese, black olives, cherry tomato halves in that order.
2. Repeat until all the ingredients are used.
3. Arrange in a serving platter.
4. Serve and enjoy!

Nutrition (Per Serving)

- Calories: 57
- Fat: 5g
- Carbohydrates: 2g
- Protein: 2g

Fluffed Up Chocolate Mousse

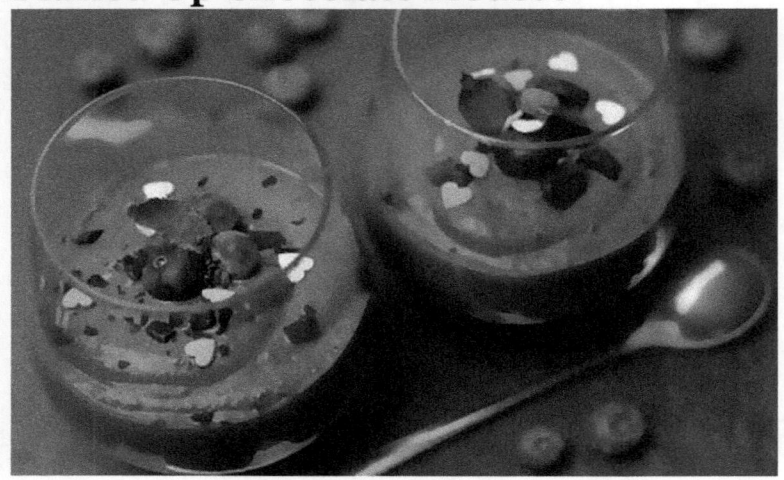

Serving: 4

Prep Time: 5 minutes

Cook Time: Nil

Ingredients

- 1 can (14.5 ounces) coconut cream, chilled
- 3 tablespoons unsweetened cocoa powder
- ¼ cup Swerve
- 1 teaspoon vanilla extract

How To

1. Take a large-sized mixing bowl and add coconut cream, whip with hand mixer.
2. Keep whipping for 3 minutes until fluffy.
3. Fold in cocoa powder, vanilla, swerve and mix.
4. Serve immediately!

Nutrition (Per Serving)

- Calories: 222
- Fat: 22g

- Carbohydrates: 4g
- Protein: 1g

Chocolate Butter Dip

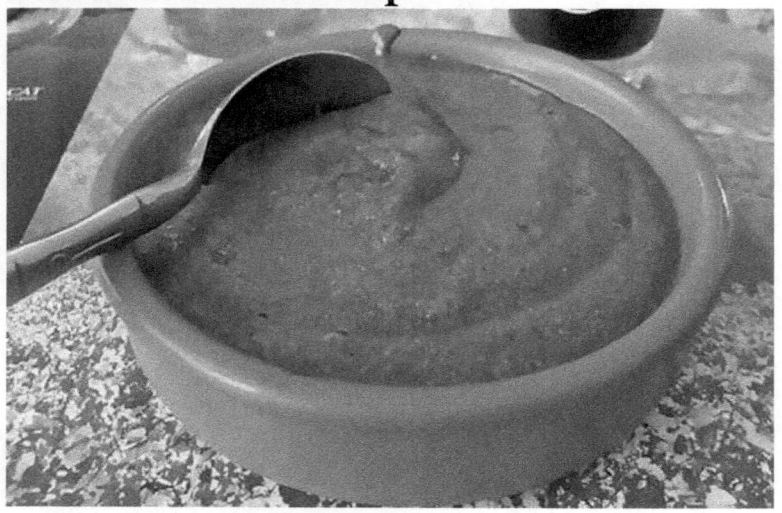

Serving: 14

Prep Time: 15 minutes

Cook Time: 0 minutes

Ingredients

- 1 cup of Plain Greek Yogurt
- ½ cup of almond butter
- 1/3 cup of chocolate hazelnut spread
- 1 tablespoon of honey
- 1 teaspoon of vanilla
- Sliced up fruits as desired, such as pears, apples, apricots, bananas, etc.

How To

1. Take a medium-sized bowl and add the first five listed ingredients.

2. With an immersion blender, blend well until you have a smooth dip.

3. Serve with your favorite sliced fruit.
4. Enjoy!

Nutrition(Per Serving)

- Calories: 115
- Fat: 8g
- Carbohydrates: 115g
- Protein: 4g

Mouthwatering Panna Cotta with Mixed Berry Compote

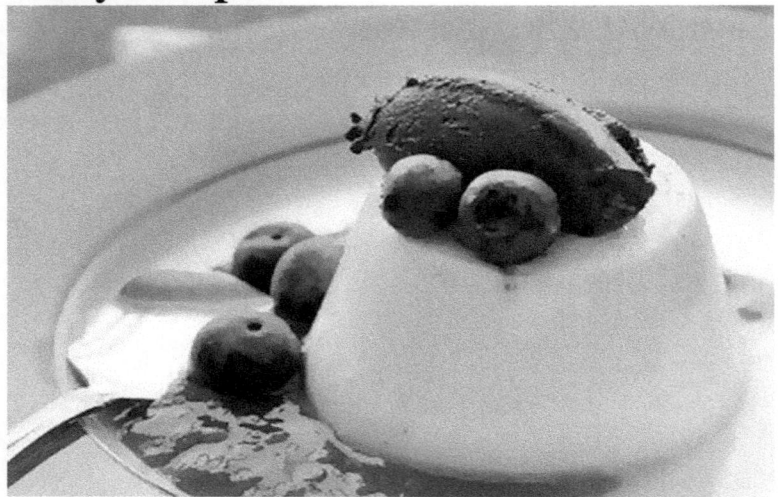

Prep Time: 5 minutes

Cooking Time: 10 minutes

Serving: 4

Ingredients

- 2 cups of freshly divided mixed berries
- 1 package of plain gelatin powder
- 1 cup of milk
- 1 2/3 cup of heavy cream
- ¾ cup of divided sugar

How To

1. Place 1 cup of raspberries into a food processor.
2. Process it to turn into a puree.
3. Take a small saucepan and transfer the puree to that saucepan.
4. Add about ¼ cup of sugar and the remaining raspberries.

5. Cook over medium heat for 10 minutes, making sure to stir from time to time.
6. Remove the heat after 10 minutes and let cool.
7. Cover and chill in your fridge.
8. Take another saucepan and combine your milk and gelatin and wait until the gelatin softens.
9. Simmer over medium heat and keep stirring frequently to fully dissolve the gelatin.
10. Stir in the heavy cream alongside the rest of the sugar and cook for another 3-5 minutes until the sugar is dissolved.
11. Pour the mixture into 4 ramekins.
12. Chill them for 8 hours or overnight.
13. Invert the mold and place on a serving plate.
14. Once the Panna Cotta comes out, top it with your berry compote.
15. Serve.

Nutrition

- Calories: 191
- Fat: 15g
- Carbohydrates: 6g
- Protein: 9g

Grilled Peaches and Egyptian Dukkah with Blueberries

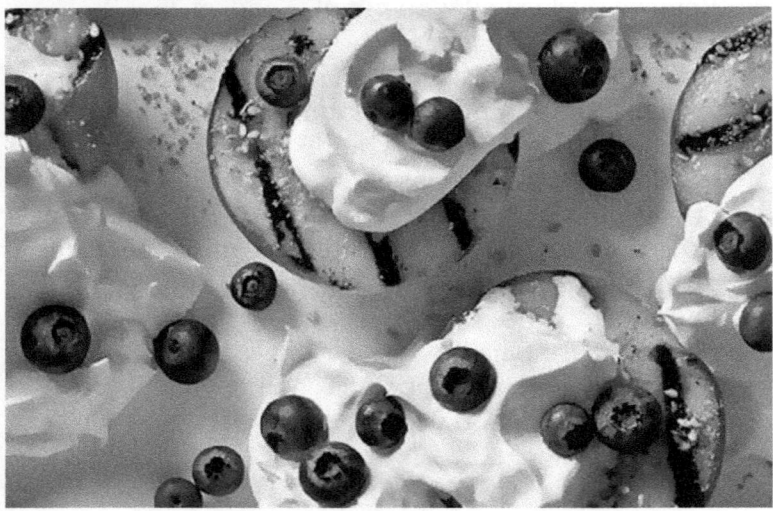

Prep Time: 5 minutes

Cooking Time: 10 minutes

Serving: 4 (1 cup of Dukkah)

Ingredients

For Dukkah

- 1/3 cup of lightly toasted pistachios
- 1/3 cup of lightly toasted almond
- 1 tablespoon of coriander seeds
- 1 tablespoon of cumin seeds
- 1 tablespoon of caraway seeds
- 1 teaspoon of crushed pepper
- 3 tablespoons of lightly toasted sesame seeds
- 2 teaspoons of fine sea salt
- 1 teaspoon of nigella seeds
- 1 teaspoon of dried mint
- 1 teaspoon of dried lemon zest

- ½ teaspoon of dried marjoram

For Peaches

- 4 pieces of peach
- Olive oil needed for brushing
- 1 tablespoon of Dukkah
- Whipped cream
- Blueberries

Process

1. For the Dukkah, first chop up your almonds and pistachios.
2. In an electric grinder or spice mill, grind up the cumin, coriander and caraway.
3. Mix all of the ingredients well in a jar.
4. Cover it tightly and set it aside.
5. If you are interested in going for direct grilling, then prepare your charcoal and gas fire first.
6. Halve and pit up the peaches.
7. Brush them up with some oil.
8. Grill the cut side down of the peaches for about 5 minutes.
9. Transfer the peaches to a plate and sprinkle some Dukkah.
10. Top with blueberries and whipped cream.
11. Serve.

Nutrition

- Calories: 204
- Fat: 18g
- Carbohydrates: 10g
- Protein: 6g

Lemon Mousse

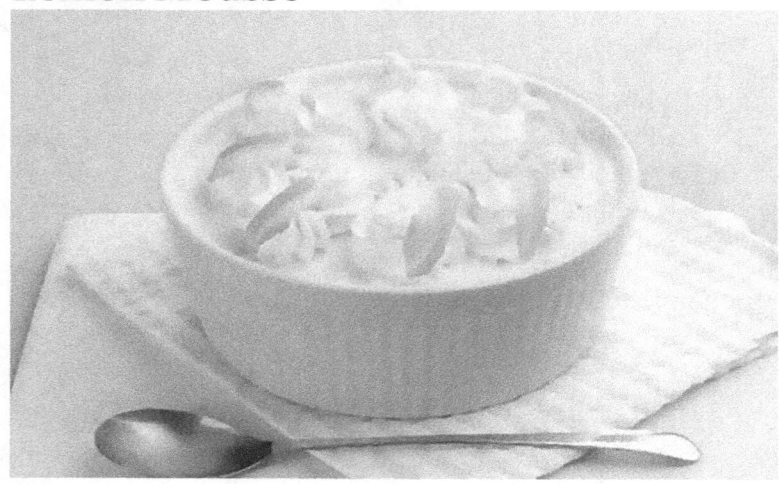

Serving: 4

Prep Time: 10 + chill time

Cook Time: 10 minutes

Ingredients

- 1 cup coconut cream
- 8 ounces cream cheese, soft
- ¼ cup fresh lemon juice
- 3 pinches salt
- 1 teaspoon lemon liquid stevia

How To

1. Pre-heat your oven to 350 degrees Fahrenheit.
2. Grease a ramekin with butter.
3. Beat cream, cream cheese, fresh lemon juice, salt and lemon liquid stevia in a mixer.
4. Pour batter into ramekin.
5. Bake for 10 minutes, then transfer mouse to serving glass.
6. Let chill for 2 hours and serve.

7. Enjoy!

Nutrition (Per Serving)

- Calories: 395
- Fat: 31g
- Carbohydrates: 3g
- Protein: 5g

Avocado Cool Dish

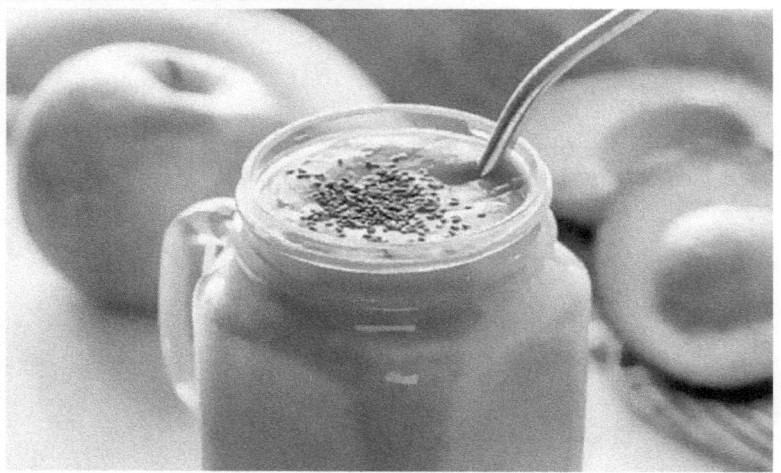

Serving: 2

Prep Time: 10 minutes

Ingredients:

- ½ avocado, cubed
- 1 cup coconut milk
- Half a lemon
- ¼ cup fresh spinach leaves
- 1 pear
- 1 tablespoon hemp seed powder

Toppings

- Handful of macadamia nuts
- Handful of grapes
- 2 lemon slices

Directions:

1. Add all the listed ingredients to your blender except coconut oil, salt and chili powder.
2. Blend until smooth.
3. Add salt, coconut oil and chili powder.

4. Stir well and serve chilled!

Nutritional Contents:

- Calories: 409
- Fat: 33g
- Carbohydrates: 8g
- Protein: 12g

Icy Berry Popsicles

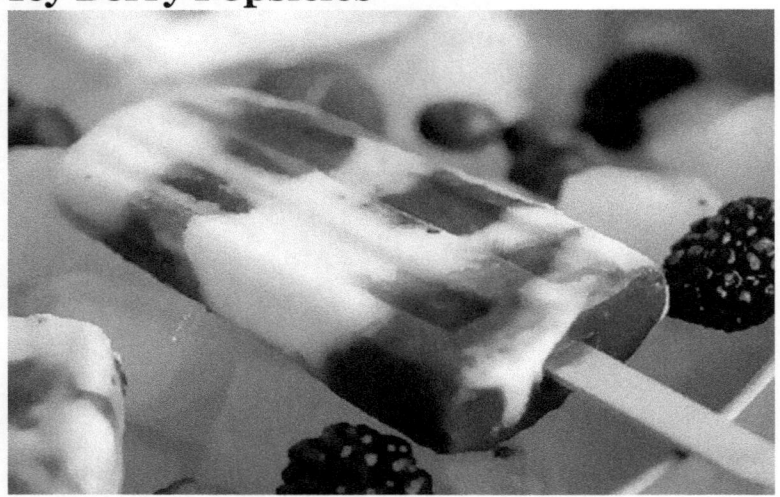

Serving: 2

Prep Time: 2 hours

Cook Time: Nil

Ingredients

- ½ can coconut cream, canned
- 2 teaspoons natural sweetener, such as stevia
- ¼ cup mixed blackberries and blueberries

How To

1. Blend the listed ingredients in a blender until smooth.
2. Pour mix into popsicle molds and let them chill for 2 hours.
3. Serve and enjoy!

Nutrition (Per Serving)

- Calories: 165
- Fat: 17g
- Carbohydrates: 2g

- Protein: 1g

Spiced Up Mug Cake

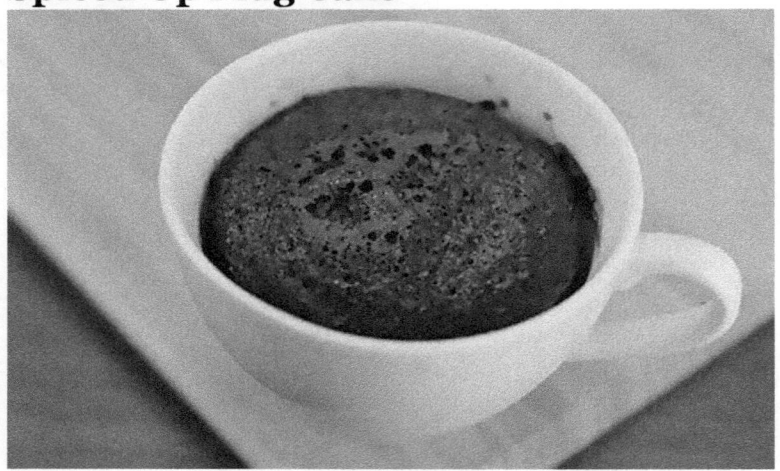

Serving: 2

Prep Time: 5 minutes

Cook Time: 5 minutes

Ingredients

- 2 tablespoons almond flour
- 1 tablespoon flaxseed meal
- 1 tablespoon butter
- 1 tablespoon cream cheese
- 1 large egg
- 1 slice bacon, cooked
- ½ jalapeno pepper
- ½ teaspoon baking powder
- ¼ teaspoon salt

How To

1. Take a frying pan and place over medium heat.
2. Add slice of bacon and cook until it has a crispy texture.
3. Mix all of the listed ingredients (including cooked bacon) into a microwave proof container, clean the sides.

4. Microwave for 75 seconds on high power.
5. Take the cup out of the microwave and tap it against a surface to take the cake out.
6. Garnish with a bit of jalapeno and serve!

<u>Nutrition (Per Serving)</u>

- Calories: 429
- Fat: 38g
- Carbohydrates: 6g
- Protein: 16g

Hearty Cashew and Almond Butter

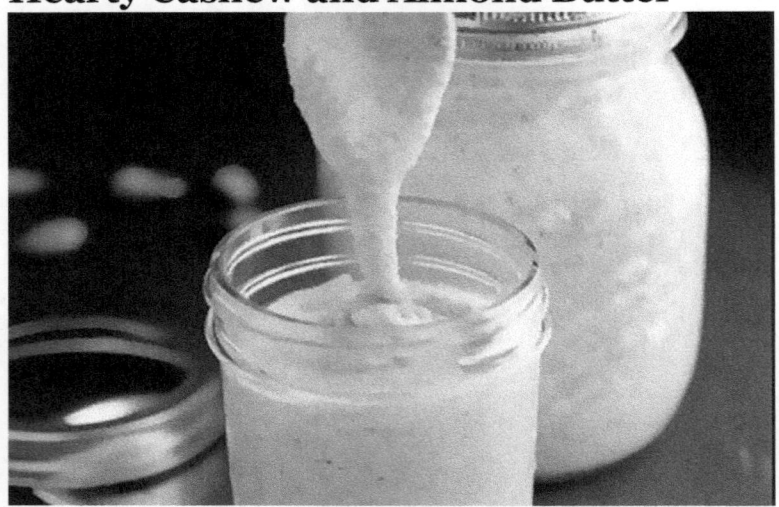

Serving: 1 and ½ cups

Prep Time: 5 minutes

Cook Time: Nil

Ingredients

- 1 cup almonds, blanched
- 1/3 cup cashew nuts
- 2 tablespoons coconut oil
- Salt as needed
- ½ teaspoon cinnamon

How To

1. Pre-heat your oven to 350 degrees Fahrenheit.
2. Bake almonds and cashews for 12 minutes.
3. Let them cool.
4. Transfer to food processor and add remaining ingredients.
5. Add oil and keep blending until smooth.
6. Serve and enjoy!

Nutrition (Per Serving)

- Calories: 205
- Fat: 19g
- Carbohydrates: g
- Protein: 2.8g

Chapter 10: Snacks
Brussels Sprouts and Pistachios

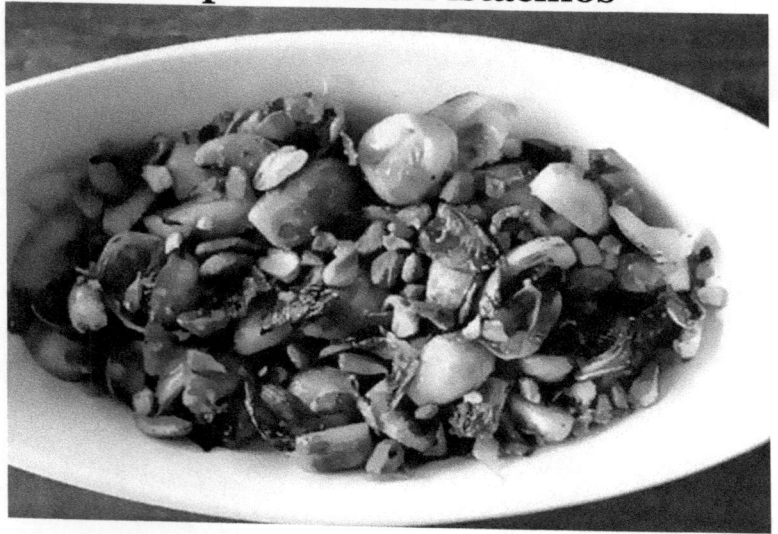

Serving: 4

Prep Time: 15 minutes

Cook Time: 15 minutes

Ingredients

- 1 pound Brussels sprouts, trimmed and halved lengthwise
- 4 shallots, peeled and quartered
- 1 tablespoon extra-virgin olive oil
- Sea salt
- Freshly ground black pepper
- ½ cup roasted pistachios, chopped
- Zest of ½ lemon
- Juice of ½ lemon

How To

1. Pre-heat your oven to 400 degrees Fahrenheit.

2. Line a baking sheet with aluminum foil and keep aside.
3. Take a large bowl and add Brussels sprouts, shallots with olive oil and coat well.
4. Season sea salt, pepper, spread veggies evenly on sheet.
5. Bake for 15 minutes until lightly caramelized.
6. Remove oven and transfer to a serving bowl.
7. Toss with lemon zest, pistachios, lemon juice.
8. Serve warm and enjoy!

Nutrition (Per Serving)

- Calories: 126
- Fat: 7g
- Carbohydrates: 14g
- Protein: 6g

Hearty Cucumber Soup

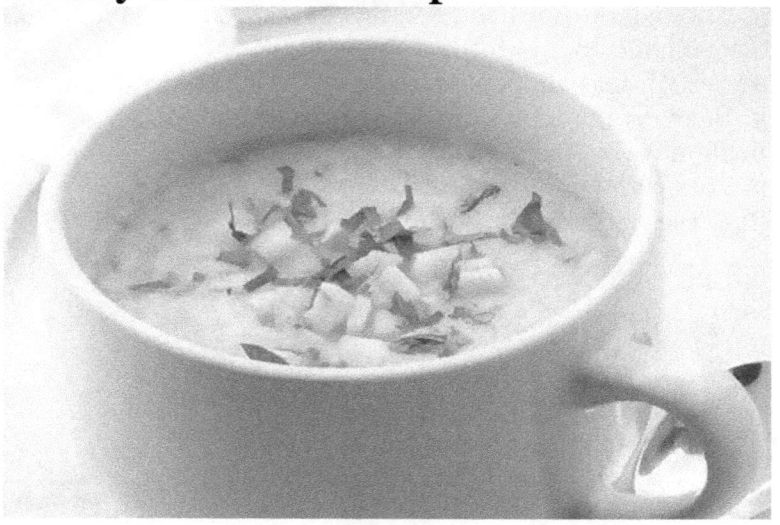

Serving: 4

Prep Time: 10 minutes

Cook Time: Nil

Ingredients

- ¼ cup Greek yogurt, plain
- ¼ cup parsley, diced
- ¼ teaspoon fried pepper flakes
- ½ whole avocado, diced
- ¼ teaspoon salt
- ½ cup veggie broth
- 1 tablespoon garlic, minced
- 2 cups cucumber, peeled and diced
- ¼ cup onions, diced
- ½ tablespoon lemon juice

How To

1. Add the listed ingredients to a blender and emulsify by blending (except ½ cup of chopped cucumbers).
2. Blend well until smooth.
3. Pour into 4 servings and top with remaining cucumbers.
4. Enjoy!

<u>Nutrition (Per Serving)</u>

- Calories: 169
- Fat: 12g
- Net Carbohydrates: 6g
- Protein: 4g

Spiced Up Kale Chips

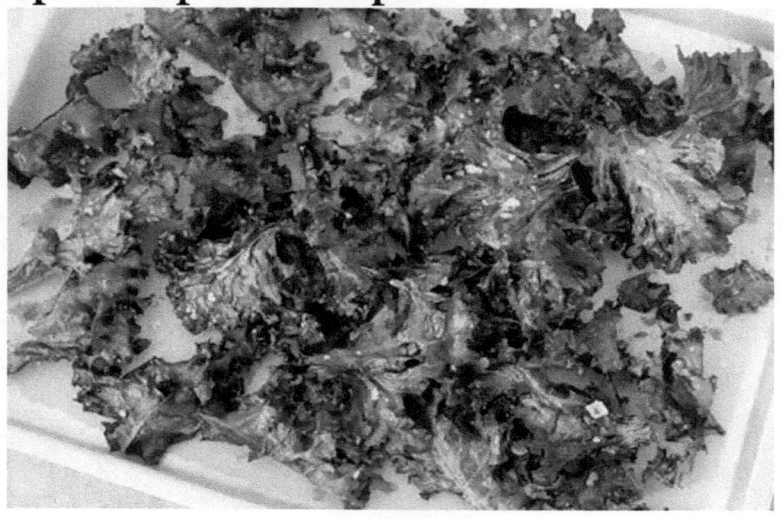

Serving: 4

Prep Time: 10 minutes

Cook Time: 25 minutes

Ingredients

- 3 cups kale, stemmed and thoroughly washed, torn into 2-inch pieces
- 1 tablespoon extra-virgin olive oil
- ½ teaspoon chili powder
- ¼ teaspoon sea salt

How To

5. Pre-heat your oven to 300 degrees Fahrenheit.
6. Line 2 baking sheets with parchment paper and keep aside.
7. Dry kale entirely and transfer to a large bowl.
8. Add olive oil and toss.
9. Make sure each leaf is covered.
10. Season kale with chili powder and salt, toss again.

11. Divide kale between baking sheets and spread into a single layer.
12. Bake for 25 minutes until crispy.
13. Cool the chips for 5 minutes and serve.
14. Enjoy!

Nutrition (Per Serving)

- Calories: 56
- Fat: 4g
- Carbohydrates: 5g
- Protein: 2g

Fresh Veggies with Hummus

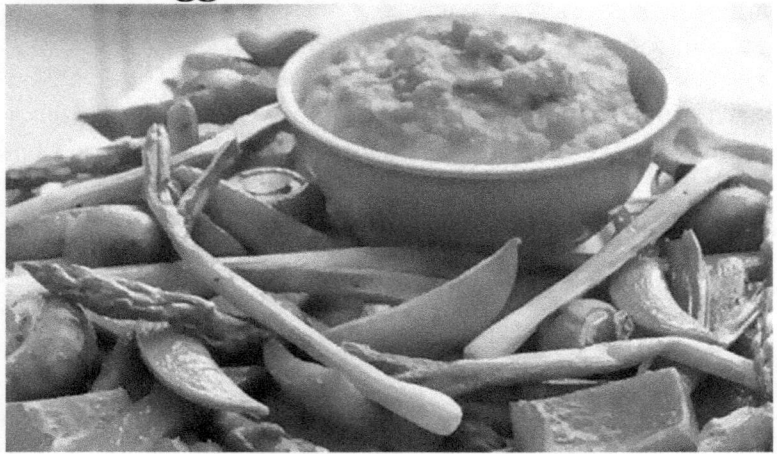

Serving: 4

Prep Time: 5 minutes

Cook Time: nil

Ingredients

- 1 can (15 ounces) chickpeas
- ¼ cup tahini
- 2 tablespoons extra virgin olive oil
- ¼ cup fresh squeezed lemon juice
- 2 garlic cloves, minced
- 2 tablespoons extra virgin olive oil
- ½ teaspoon ground cumin
- ¾ cup fire roasted red peppers
- Pinch of cayenne pepper
- Assorted selection of veggies such as cauliflower, broccoli florets, carrot sticks, snow peas, celery

How To

1. Add all of the listed ingredients (except veggies) and blend until you have a nice consistency.

2. Serve the hummus with raw veggies.
3. Enjoy!

Nutrition (Per Serving)

- Calories: 50
- Fat: 4g
- Carbohydrates: 4g
- Protein: 1g

Crazy Almond Crackers

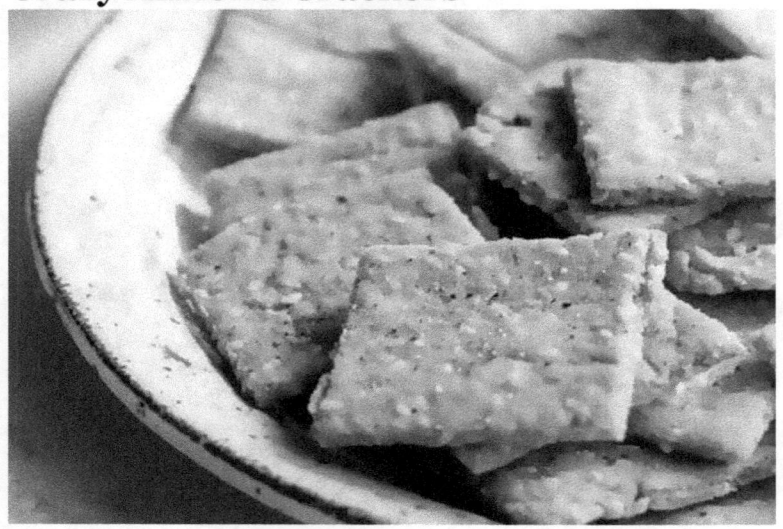

Serving: 40 crackers

Prep Time: 10 minutes

Cook Time: 20 minutes

Ingredients

- 1 cup almond flour
- ¼ teaspoon baking soda
- ¼ teaspoon salt
- 1/8 teaspoon black pepper
- 3 tablespoons sesame seeds
- 1 egg, beaten
- Salt and pepper to taste

How To

1. Pre-heat your oven to 350 degrees Fahrenheit.
2. Line two baking sheets with parchment paper and keep aside.
3. Mix the dry ingredients to a large bowl and add egg, mix well and form dough.

4. Divide dough into two balls.
5. Roll out the dough between two pieces of parchment paper.
6. Cut into crackers and transfer them to prepared baking sheet.
7. Bake for 15-20 minutes.
8. Repeat until all the dough has been used up.
9. Leave crackers to cool and serve.
10. Enjoy!

Nutrition (Per Serving)

- Calories: 302
- Fat: 28g
- Carbohydrates: 4g
- Protein: 9g

Superb Stuffed Mushrooms

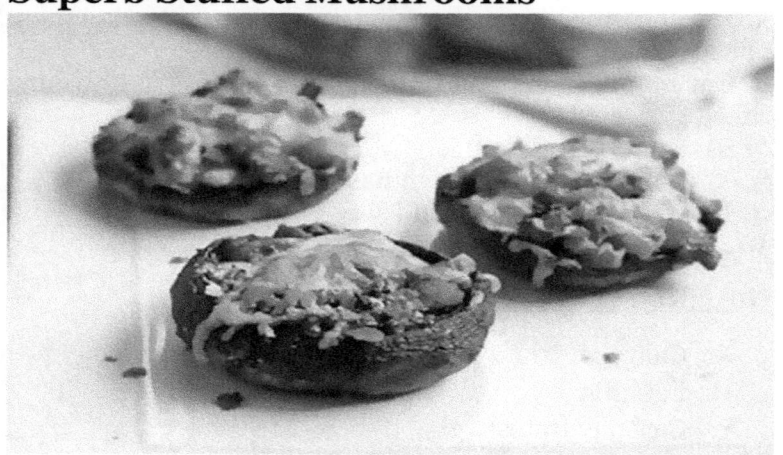

Serving: 4

Prep Time: 10 minutes

Cook Time: 15 minutes

Ingredients

- 4 Portobello mushrooms
- 1 cup crumbled blue cheese
- 2 teaspoons extra virgin olive oil
- Salt, to taste
- Fresh thyme

How To

1. Preheat your oven to 350 degree Fahrenheit.
2. Cut out the stems from the mushrooms.
3. Chop them into small pieces.
4. Take a bowl and mix stem pieces with thyme, salt and blue cheese and mix well.
5. Fill up mushroom with the prepared cheese.
6. Top with some oil.
7. Take a baking sheet and place the mushrooms.

8. Bake for 15 minutes to 20 minutes.
9. Serve warm and enjoy!

Nutrition (Per Serving)

- Calories: 124
- Fat: 22.4g
- Carbohydrates: 5.4g
- Protein: 1.2g

Flax and Almond Crunchies

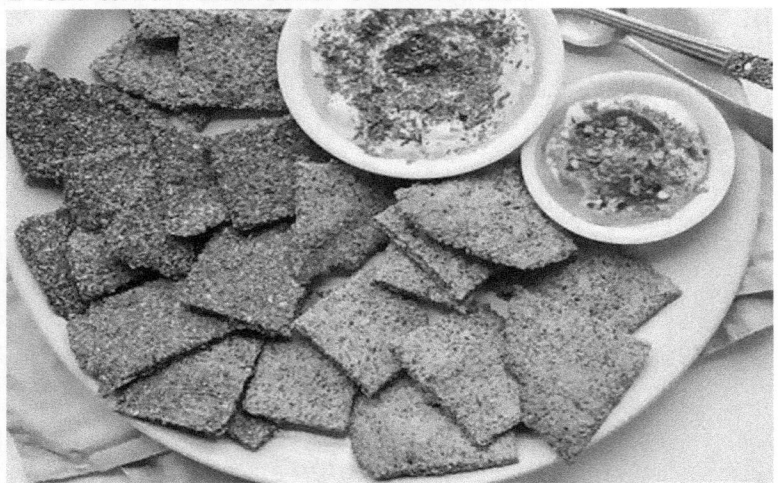

Serving: 20 Crackers

Prep Time: 15 minutes

Cook Time: 60 minutes

Ingredients

- ½ cup ground flax seeds
- ½ cup almond flour
- 1 tablespoon coconut flour
- 2 tablespoons shelled hemp seeds
- ¼ teaspoon sea salt, plus more to sprinkle on top
- 1 egg white
- 2 tablespoons unsalted butter, melted

How To

1. Pre-heat your oven to 300 degrees Fahrenheit.
2. Take a baking sheet and line it with parchment paper, keep the prepared sheet on the side.
3. Add flax, coconut flour, almond, salt, hemp seed to a bowl and mix well.
4. Add egg and melted butter, mix well.

5. Transfer dough to sheet of parchment paper and cover with another sheet of paper.
6. Roll out dough.
7. Cut into crackers and bake for 60 minutes.
8. Cool and serve!

Nutrition (Per Serving)

- Calories: 47
- Fat: 6g
- Carbohydrates: 1.2g
- Protein: 02g

Mashed Up Celeriac

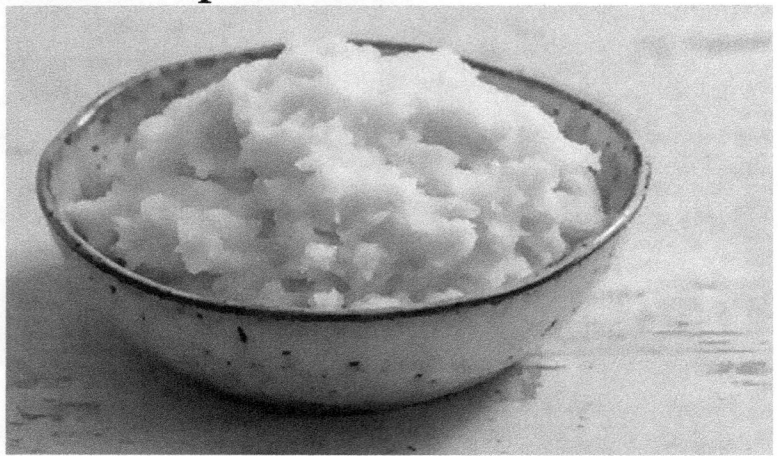

Serving: 4

Prep Time: 10 minutes

Cook Time: 20 minutes

Ingredients

- 2 celeriac, washed, peeled and diced
- 2 teaspoons extra-virgin olive oil
- 1 tablespoon honey
- ½ teaspoon ground nutmeg
- Sea salt
- Freshly ground black pepper

How To

1. Pre-heat your oven to 400 degrees Fahrenheit.
2. Line a baking sheet with aluminum foil and keep it aside.
3. Take a large bowl and toss celeriac and olive oil.
4. Spread celeriac evenly on baking sheet.
5. Roast for 20 minutes until tender.
6. Transfer to large bowl.
7. Add honey and nutmeg.

8. Use a potato masher to mash the mixture until fluffy.
9. Season with salt and pepper.
10. Serve and enjoy!

Nutrition (Per Serving)

- Calories: 136
- Fat: 3g
- Carbohydrates: 26g
- Protein: 4g

Baked Feta and Spinach Meal

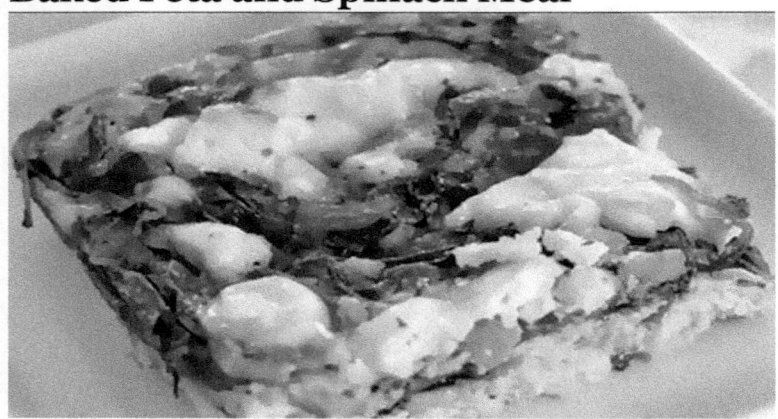

Serving: 6

Prep Time: 10 minutes

Cook Time: 12 minutes

Ingredients

- 6 ounces sun-dried tomato pesto
- 6 (6 inch) whole wheat pita bread
- 2 Roma plum tomatoes, chopped
- 1 bunch rinsed spinach, chopped
- 4 fresh mushrooms, sliced
- ½ cup feta cheese, crumbled
- 2 tablespoons Parmesan cheese, crumbled
- 3 tablespoons olive oil
- Ground black pepper

How To

1. Pre-heat your oven to a temperature of 350 degree Fahrenheit.
2. Spread your tomato pesto onto one side of your pita bread and place on your baking sheet (with the pesto side up).

3. Top the pitas with spinach, tomatoes, feta cheese, mushrooms and Parmesan cheese.
4. Drizzle with some olive oil and season nicely with pepper.
5. Bake in your oven for about 12 minutes until the breads are crispy.
6. Cut up the pita into quarters and serve!

Nutrition (Per Serving)

- Calories: 350
- Fat: 17g
- Carbohydrates: 41g
- Protein: 11g

Easy Medi Kale

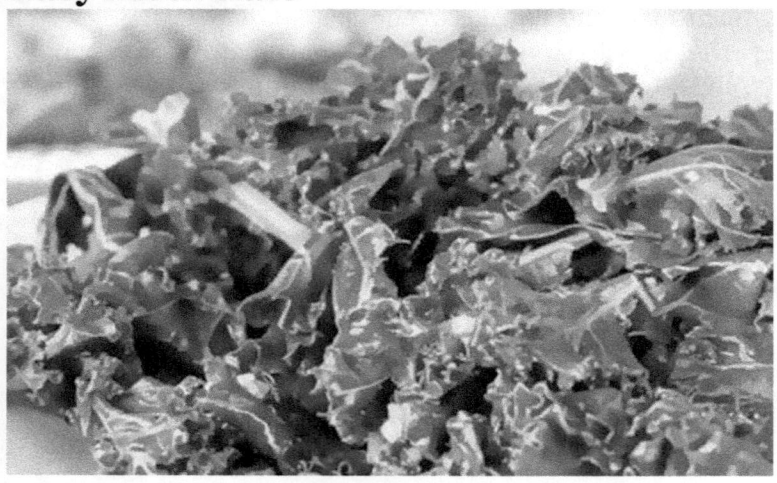

Serving: 6

Prep Time: 15 minutes

Cook Time: 10 minutes

Ingredients

- 12 cups kale, chopped
- 2 tablespoons lemon juice
- 1 tablespoon olive oil
- 1 tablespoon garlic, minced
- 1 teaspoon soy sauce
- Salt and pepper as needed

How To

1. Add a steamer insert to your saucepan.
2. Fill the saucepan with water up to the bottom of the steamer.
3. Cover and bring water to boil (medium-high heat).
4. Add kale to the insert and steam for 7-8 minutes.
5. Take a large bowl and add lemon juice, garlic, olive oil, salt, soy sauce and pepper.

6. Mix well and add the steamed kale to the bowl.
7. Toss and serve.
8. Enjoy!

Nutrition (Per Serving)

- Calories: 350
- Fat: 17g
- Carbohydrates: 41g
- Protein: 11g

Black Bean Hummus

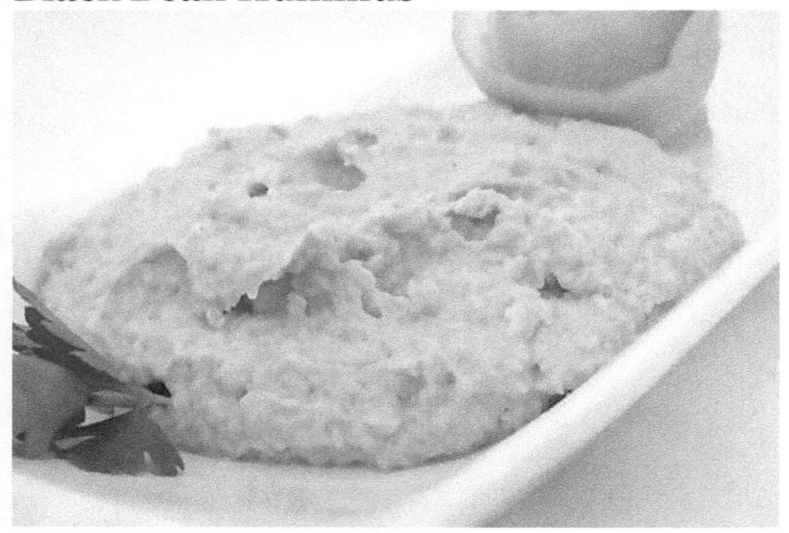

Serving: 4

Prep Time: 25 minutes

Cook Time: 0 minute

Ingredients

- 1 cup of cooked black beans
- 1 minced garlic clove
- 2 tablespoons of olive oil
- 2 tablespoons of lemon juice
- 1 tablespoon of white wine vinegar
- ½ teaspoon of ground cumin
- Salt and pepper as needed
- ½ a head of iceberg lettuce cut up into wedges

How To

1. Add all the listed ingredients to your blender (except lettuce).
2. Process until everything is smooth.

3. Allow to sit for 15 minutes and serve with the iceberg lettuce.
4. Enjoy!

Nutrition(Per Serving)

- Calories: 81
- Fat: 4g
- Carbohydrates: 10g
- Protein: 4g

Strawberry and Feta Salad

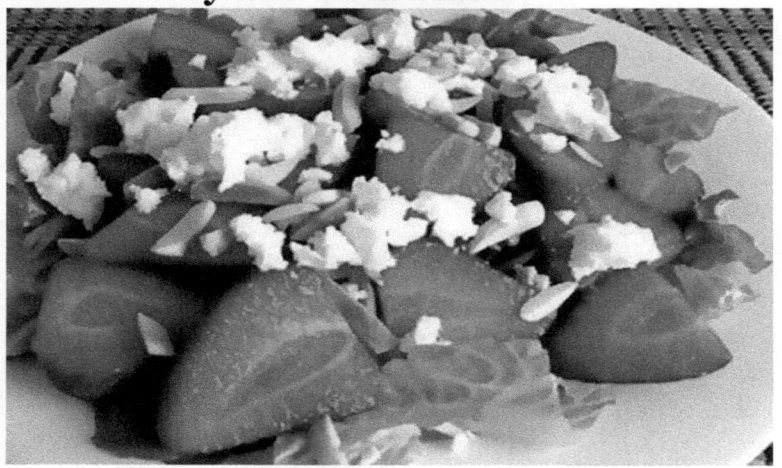

Prep Time: 10 minutes

Cooking Time: 0 minutes

Serving: 4

Ingredients

- 4 cups of baby spinach
- 6 ounces of crumbled feta cheese
- 1 cup of thinly sliced fresh strawberries
- ½ cup of chopped walnuts
- Balsamic-Dijon Vinaigrette
- 2 tablespoons of extra virgin olive oil
- 2 tablespoons of balsamic vinegar
- 1 tablespoon of Dijon mustard
- 1 tablespoon of honey
- Salt as needed
- Pepper as needed

How To

1. Take a small-sized glass bowl and mix in the olive oil, Dijon mustard, balsamic vinegar and honey.

2. Season with some pepper and salt.
3. Toss the spinach, strawberries, feta, walnuts and pine nuts in a large sized mixing bowl.
4. Divide the mixture amongst serving plates and dress with the previously prepared vinaigrette dressing.
5. Serve.

Nutrition

- Calories: 270
- Fat: 22g
- Carbohydrates: 11g
- Protein: 9g

Baked Falafel Dish

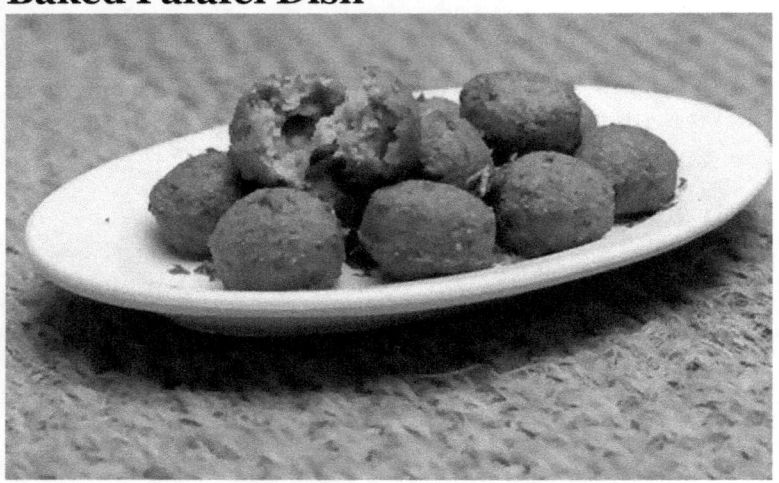

Serving: 2

Prep Time: 20 minutes

Cook Time: 20 minutes

Ingredients

- ¼ cup of chopped onion
- 15 ounces of garbanzo beans rinsed and drained
- 3 minced garlic cloves
- ¼ cup of chopped fresh parsley
- 1 teaspoon of ground cumin
- ¼ teaspoon of ground coriander
- ¼ teaspoon of salt
- ¼ teaspoon of baking soda
- 1 tablespoon of all-purpose flour
- 1 beaten egg
- 2 tablespoons of olive oil

How To

1. Wrap the onion in cheese cloth and squeeze as much moisture as possible, keep it aside.

2. Take a food processor and add beans, parsley, garlic, coriander, cumin, baking soda and salt.
3. Blitz well and transfer the mixture to the onion.
4. Stir in eggs, flour and mix well.
5. Shape the mixture into patties and allow to stand for 15 minutes.
6. Pre-heat your oven to 400 degrees Fahrenheit.
7. Take a skillet and place it over medium-high heat
8. Heat some oil.
9. Add your prepared patties to your skillet and cook for about 3 minutes on each side until browned.
10. Transfer them to your pre-heated oven, bake for about 10 minutes and serve!

Nutrition(Per Serving)

- Calories: 281
- Fat: 10g
- Carbohydrates: 39g
- Protein: 11g

Conclusion

I would like to thank you for purchasing the book and taking the time to go through it.

I do hope that this book has been helpful, and you found the information contained within the recipes useful!

Keep in mind that you are not only limited to the recipes provided in this book! Just keep exploring until you create your very own Mediterranean Magnum opus!

Stay healthy and stay safe!

© Copyright 2019 – Tina Cooper- All rights reserved.

In no way is it legal to reproduce, duplicate, or transmit any part of this document by either electronic means or in printed format. Recording of this publication is strictly prohibited, and any storage of this material is not allowed unless with written permission from the publisher. All rights reserved.

The information provided herein is stated to be truthful and consistent, in that any liability, regarding inattention or otherwise, by any usage or abuse of any policies, processes, or directions contained within is the solitary and complete responsibility of the recipient reader. Under no circumstances will any legal liability or blame be held against the publisher for any reparation, damages, or monetary loss due to the information herein, either directly or indirectly.

Respective authors own all copyrights not held by the publisher.

Legal Notice:

This book is copyright protected. This is only for personal use. You cannot amend, distribute, sell, use, quote or paraphrase any part or the content within this book without the consent of the author or copyright owner. Legal action will be pursued if this is breached.

Disclaimer Notice:

Please note the information contained within this document is for educational and entertainment purposes only. Every attempt has been made to provide accurate, up to date and reliable, complete information. No warranties of any kind are expressed or implied. Readers acknowledge that the author is not engaging in the rendering of legal, financial, medical or professional advice.

By reading this document, the reader agrees that under no circumstances are we responsible for any losses, direct or indirect, which are incurred as a result of the use of information contained in this document, including, but not limited to, —errors, omissions, or inaccuracies.